The 7 Step Diabetes Fitness Plan

"The important message from this book is that losing weight may not be the panacea it was once thought to be for people with type 2 diabetes. In fact, becoming fit may have a greater effect on your blood glucose control than losing weight. And only exercise seems to be able to reduce the amount of internal stomach fat that is the most dangerous kind.

"This should come as good news to the many type 2 diabetes patients who have extreme difficulty losing weight (especially when given diabetes drugs that cause weight gain) and who suffer from constant nagging from health care workers who tell them to 'just lose a little weight and your diabetes will go away.'

"Colberg, an exercise physiologist, explains this in detail and then gives useful tips on how to work more exercise into your daily regime, how to exercise, and how to stay motivated to exercise."

—GRETCHEN BECKER,
author of *The First Year—Type 2 Diabetes* and
Prediabetes: What You Need to Know to Keep Diabetes Away

"*The 7 Step Diabetes Fitness Plan* is a must for all people with type 2 diabetes who want to take control of their disease. While the focus of the book is on exercise, it provides both an excellent review of what's known about what causes diabetes as well as a great review of dietary and psychological factors that impact on it. Its practical program of diet and physical exercise will help everyone who has diabetes or is at risk for diabetes improve their health."

—RICHARD S. SURWIT, PhD,
Duke University Medical Center,
author of *The Mind-Body Diabetes Revolution*

About the Author

Sheri R. Colberg, PhD, is an exercise physiologist and associate professor of exercise science at Old Dominion University in Norfolk, Virginia. Having earned an undergraduate degree from Stanford University and a PhD from University of California, Berkeley, she specializes in all aspects of diabetes and exercise, including clinical research on type 2 diabetes and exercise funded by the American Diabetes Association (ADA). She has also authored more than sixty articles and two other books: *The Diabetic Athlete* (Human Kinetics, 2001) and *Diabetes-Free Kids* (Avery, June 2005).

In addition to her many professional credentials, which include being an exercise specialist in a diabetes treatment center, Dr. Colberg has almost four decades–worth of practical experience living well and being fit as a (type 1) diabetic exerciser. She lectures frequently across the nation and is also a reviewer for many scientific journals, a member of several diabetes advisory/editorial boards and an online diabetes resource (dLife.com), a fellow of the American College of Sports Medicine, and an ADA professional member. She also has been quoted frequently by the media in national magazines and on television, radio, and the Internet.

An avid recreational exerciser, Dr. Colberg resides in Virginia Beach, Virginia with her husband and their three boys. Please visit her Web site at www.SheriColberg.com or e-mail her at Sheri@SheriColberg.com.

The 7 Step Diabetes Fitness Plan

The **7** Step Diabetes Fitness Plan

Living Well and Being Fit with Diabetes,
No Matter Your Weight

Sheri R. Colberg, PhD

FOREWORD BY ANNE PETERS, MD

MARLOWE & COMPANY
NEW YORK

THE 7 STEP DIABETES FITNESS PLAN:
Living Well and Being Fit with Diabetes, No Matter Your Weight

Copyright © 2006 by Sheri R. Colberg
Foreword copyright© 2006 by Anne Peters, MD
Exercise illustrations copyright © 2006 by Patrick Ochs

Published by
Marlowe & Company
An Imprint of Avalon Publishing Group Incorporated

AVALON

Library of Congress Cataloging-in-Publication Data
Colberg, Sheri, 1963–
The 7 step diabetes fitness plan : living well and being fit with diabetes, no
matter your weight / Sheri R. Colberg ; foreword by Anne Peters.
p. cm.
Includes bibliographical references and index.
ISBN 1-56924-331-X (pbk.)
1. Diabetics—Rehabilitation. 2. Chronic diseases--Exercise therapy.
3. Diabetes—Treatment. 4. Physical fitness.
I. Title: Seven step diabetes fitness plan. II. Title.
RC661.E94C65 2006
616.4'62062--dc22
2005026993

ISBN 13: 978-1-56924-331-2

DESIGNED BY PAULINE NEUWIRTH, NEUWIRTH & ASSOCIATES, INC.

Printed in the United States of America

In loving memory of my grandmother, Velda Huffman Stubbs,

who good-heartedly tolerated my attempts to make her into a

fit diabetic when I was only a precocious preteen.

Contents

Foreword

Anne Peters, MD

M Y LIFE IS devoted to taking care of people who are at risk for dia-betes as well as those who already have diabetes. My patients come in all shapes and sizes, ethnicities, and ages. Some have been diag-nosed recently; others have been dealing with their diabetes and its challenges for many years. I see people I can help and, sadly, others whose complications from diabetes are too far advanced. Increasingly I see patients who are asking how to avoid getting diabetes and I rejoice in this trend. To be able to stop this disease before it begins is one of the joys of my life. I see overweight and sedentary middle-aged men and women who wrestle daily to change their diet and exercise habits so they won't suffer from complications of diabetes, such as blindness or life on dial-ysis. On the same day that I see a fifty-six-year-old double amputee in a wheelchair, I may also see a seventy-six-year-old who's had diabetes since the 1940s who never misses his daily four-mile walk with his dog. I know that for each and every one of these people, diabetes complica-tions can be minimized or prevented altogether. I laid out the path to doing so in my own book, *Conquering Diabetes* (Hudson Street Press, 2005); now Dr. Colberg gives you a complementary route to succeed-ing in accomplishing these same worthy goals.

As an exercise physiologist, Dr. Colberg's focus is more on physical activity than mine as a diabetes physician is. In fact, she is the person I turn to when I need to know more about how to treat an athlete. Having accompanied my swimmer, Gary Hall Jr., to the Sydney and Athens Olympics (and helping him win six medals, three of them gold!) I am often sought out as an expert on diabetes and exercise. But truth be told, Dr. Colberg is my expert, and now she can also be yours.

Personally, I dislike exercise. Every second I am exercising, I am thinking about how soon I can stop. My brain is engaged in a continuous conflict between my desire to quit and my commitment to stay fit. Since it is always a struggle, you'd think I'd give it up. But do you know what I hate even more than exercising? Being out of shape. I hate how I feel if I don't exercise. And although I dislike the act of exercising, I am always glad that I've done it.

I am definitely not a saint about exercising regularly. There are weeks in which I can exercise only once or twice, and there are weeks, occasionally, when I go on strike because my body needs a break. But the following week I'm back to the routine. Perhaps the most valuable lesson about fitness that we can all learn from Dr. Colberg is how to fit more physical activity into our daily lives so naturally we don't even realize we're doing it. For example, on an average day at the clinic, I put in close to ten thousand steps just going from patient to patient—so I'm not doing as badly as I thought. When I do find time to fit in my more formal exercise routine, I'm just enhancing my fitness level that much more.

Diabetes is growing at an epidemic rate, in the United States and worldwide. According to the most recent statistics, from 2000, one out of every three children born in the United States will develop diabetes in their lifetime. This number increases to one in two if the child is Latino or African American. What's traditionally been known as "adult-onset" diabetes is being diagnosed at younger and younger ages. If a person is diagnosed with diabetes at age twenty, that person can count on seventeen fewer years of life compared to a person without diabetes. Seventeen years. It could mean you won't live long enough to retire, or play with your grandchildren, or celebrate your thirty-fifth wedding anniversary. Even if you get diabetes later in life, say at age sixty, nine years of your life will be lost. But the good news is that if you take good care of your diabetes, you don't have to miss out on these and other wonderful experiences due to complications that are—and I can't stress this enough—preventable.

So, why wait until you have diabetes—or irreversible health complications that limit your quality of life—before you do anything about it? It is no longer enough to sit back and let your physician tell you what to do. Each of us must become empowered health-care consumers. Medicine is changing rapidly, and sometimes even doctors have trouble keeping up. Many people take their health for granted until they become ill, when it is often too late for doctors to make a big difference anyway. Dr. Colberg's 7 *Step Diabetes Fitness Plan* will not only help those who have diabetes to live well with it, it will help those who don't have it from developing it in the first place. It's never too soon to take your life (and your health) into your own hands and to live well, become fit, and enjoy a longer, healthier life.

Anne Peters, MD, one of the top twenty physicians treating diabetes in America, is director of the University of Southern California clinical diabetes programs and professor at the USC Keck School of Medicine. She is also currently the physician in charge of developing the nation's largest outreach program for community-based diabetes prevention and treatment. Her research has been published in such leading medical journals as the *Journal of the American Medical Association,* the *Annals of Internal Medicine,* the *American Journal of Medicine,* and *Diabetes Care.*

Ignorance Is Not Bliss

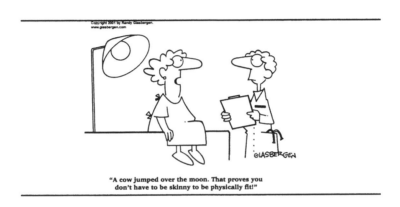

"A cow jumped over the moon. That proves you
don't have to be skinny to be physically fit!"

AMERICANS ARE UNDENIABLY getting heavier by the minute. Maybe you also find yourself lamenting about your ever-increasing body weight, but wonder if all that extra **fat** means that your health will invariably suffer. The answer is that it depends. Many people who put on too much fat also suffer from other health problems, including **diabetes**. In fact, a diabetes epidemic is currently sweeping the nation—and the world.

More than 90 percent of people developing diabetes are developing **type 2 diabetes**, characterized primarily by **insulin resistance**, or an inability of the **hormone** called **insulin** to work effectively to keep blood sugars (referred to throughout this book as **blood glucose,** or **BG**) in check. Although a minority, the people with **type 1 diabetes**, which is caused by their bodies' own destruction of insulin-producing **beta cells** in the **pancreas** (essentially **autoimmunity** triggered by an environmental cause), can also develop an insulin-resistant state that makes their diabetes harder to control. Of late, a new type of diabetes—unofficially known as **type 1.5 diabetes,** or "double diabetes"—has been emerging; it has characteristics of both type 1 (autoimmunity) and type 2 (insulin resistance) diabetes, making it difficult to make an accurate initial diagnosis in all cases.

If you are reading this book, that means either diabetes or a pre-diabetic condition (characterized primarily by insulin resistance, with a closer-to-normal BG level) has already happened to you or someone you know or care about. Perhaps your doctor recently told you that you have type 2 diabetes, which is frequently diagnosed by a **fasting** BG level of 126 milligrams per deciliter (**mg/dl**) or above first thing in the morning, or perhaps your sugars have been hovering in the prediabetic range (100 to 125 mg/dl prebreakfast) as your body weight has been creeping up. You may want to blame the half-dozen glazed doughnuts or that triple-fudge sundae you just ate, instead of diabetes or **predia-betes** for a passing BG reading of 200 mg/dl, but you can't. The reality is that regardless of what you eat, your BG level will never spike above 140 mg/dl if you don't already have one of these health conditions.

A doctor may have already advised you to lose some weight to better control your BG, but is losing weight the only solution? If it is, then most people are out of luck. The reality is that only a fraction of the millions of dieters—with or without diabetes—succeed in losing weight and keeping it off permanently. Obesity and diabetes are currently overtaking our nation. Two-thirds of American adults are considered **over-weight** or **obese,** and that number is rising fast, particularly among younger adults and youth, based on their **body mass index** (**BMI**).

Even more alarming is the fact that children born nowadays have a one-in-three chance of developing diabetes in their lifetime, and for many minority groups, the risk is close to a whopping 50 percent. More than 20.8 million people in the United States already have diabetes, and the projected number of Americans with diabetes by 2030 is over 30 million. That's an overwhelming number of Americans with diabetes, and that doesn't even include the more than 40 million insulin-resistant, pre-diabetic people who have a strong potential for developing it. Moreover, among the nearly 370 million cases of diabetes projected worldwide by 2030 (up from 170 million in 2000), the United States lags behind only India and China, two countries with much larger populations.

Why should you worry about diabetes?

As many as a third of the people who have diabetes don't even know it. So, is ignorance bliss? Absolutely not, because you can't fight back against diabetes—or even prediabetes—unless you're aware of your condition and ready to do something about it. Having diabetes is definitely something to worry about.

Diabetes has the potential not only to rob you of, on average, more than 12 years of your life, it can also dramatically reduce your quality of life for more than 20 years. Diabetes can result in compromised physical capacity, partial limb amputations, loss of mobility, chronic pain, blindness, chronic **dialysis**, and **heart disease**. For women, the reality may be even worse: 38.5 percent of average females born in the year 2000 or later are predicted to develop diabetes; diabetes will cut short the lives of these women by 14.3 years if they are diagnosed by the age of forty and lower their quality of life for 22 of the years they do live.

Our current national health problems are irrefutably serious. In fact, the generation of Americans now being born is the first ever predicted to die before their parents. If you or your kids have diabetes, you have twice the risk of dying compared to anyone without the disease, and if you're younger when diagnosed with diabetes (age twenty-five to forty-four), your risk is almost four times as high as your nondiabetic counterparts. Diabetes is the sixth leading cause of death in the United States, based on death certificates listing it as the cause. However, these statistics belie its significant negative impact on longevity, as many death certificates list diabetes only as a contributing cause of death; still more fail to mention it at all. For instance, if someone with diabetes dies from a **heart attack**, the death certificate may not even list diabetes as a cause or contributor, even though it is well documented that poor control of BG levels accelerates the blockage of **coronary** arteries, which leads to heart disease. A newly released study from the World Health Organization found that diabetes kills more people worldwide than was previously suspected: it is currently the cause of 3.2 million deaths per year, or 6 deaths every minute.

Heart disease is the leading cause of death in people with diabetes. In fact, if you have diabetes, you now have the same risk of having a heart attack as someone without diabetes but with known heart disease who has already had at least one coronary event. Many undiagnosed people with type 2 diabetes actually first learn of their condition shortly after having their first heart attack. It's likely that they have already had undetected diabetes for a number of years, long enough for it to cause significant damage. **Plaque** buildup in the coronary arteries begins in childhood. In adulthood, the heart disease process continues, and when commonly coexisting health issues such as high blood pressure and elevated blood fats are also present, plaque formation is further accelerated. Moreover, almost three-fourths of adults with diabetes have high blood pressure (an average reading of above 130 over 90), which may or may not be effectively controlled with medications. Insulin resistance itself may be even more important to control than BG levels to reduce your risk of a heart disease.

Diabetes is also well known for its damaging effects on the eyes, kidneys, and nerves, which can significantly lower quality of life. Poorly controlled diabetes is the leading cause of new cases of blindness among adults, and proliferative diabetic **retinopathy** (one form of diabetic eye disease) alone causes tens of thousands of new cases of blindness each year. In addition, diabetes causes six other eye diseases, including glaucoma, cataracts, and **neuropathy** of the optic or eye muscle nerves. Diabetes is the leading cause of new cases of end-stage kidney disease, treatable in the short term with dialysis and in the long term only with kidney transplants. As for damage to the nervous system, 60 to 70 percent of diabetic individuals have mild to severe nerve damage, including impaired sensation (numbness) in their feet or hands, **gastroparesis** (slowing of the digestion of food), carpal tunnel syndrome, **hypoglycemic unawareness** (loss of ability to sense low BG levels), and **orthostatic hypotension** (severe dizziness when standing up). The majority of toe, foot, and lower limb amputations, or more than 40,000 amputations annually, also occur among people with diabetes. As if all this weren't enough, diabetes is also the cause of increased incidence of periodontal (gum) disease and the greater incidence of birth defects in infants born to mothers with poorly controlled BG levels.

The point of discussing the more negative aspects of diabetes is not to depress or scare you, but rather to convince you that your primary goal should be to prevent, reverse, or effectively control insulin resistance and BG levels so that you can prevent these complications from ever happening to you. The good news is that they are almost entirely preventable with good BG control. An added bonus is that the majority of the same strategies used to control diabetes and its complications will also reverse a prediabetic state and potentially prevent diabetes from ever happening to you in the first place.

The problem with current diabetes care, however, is that most people never achieve or maintain optimal control over their BG levels ("optimal" means average BG in a normal or near-normal range, or a **glycated hemoglobin** level of no more than 7 percent). In fact, according to a recent report, only 37 percent of people in the United States with diagnosed diabetes ever achieve this level of control, and as many as a third of the others are still unaware of their condition and the damage it is already causing to their bodies.

All is not lost

Can you live a long and healthy life with diabetes? Certainly, and this book will teach you the steps to take to do so. After reading this book, you will also understand better why losing a significant amount of your excess pounds is not the cure-all it was once believed to be. Yes, it is possible to be fit but still overweight and to live well with diabetes (or prediabetes).

Now I'd like you to get up, stretch, and walk around for a bit (actually, I'd like you to repeat this between every fitness step); then, come back and read on to learn the seven steps to diabetes fitness. (A handy recap of all seven steps can be found in Appendix A, at the back of the book.) You will learn all you need to know to become more fit in every sense of the word, and to live a longer, healthier life without dieting—and in spite of having diabetes.

The **7** Step
Diabetes
Fitness
Plan

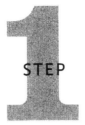

STEP 1

Get Down to Basics

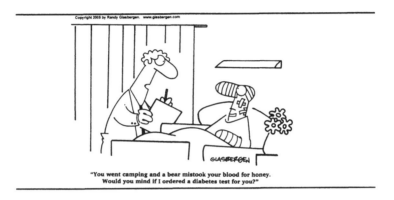

"You went camping and a bear mistook your blood for honey.
Would you mind if I ordered a diabetes test for you?"

How did you get diabetes or prediabetes in the first place? For me, this question is easy to answer: I had the mumps virus at four years of age and was diagnosed with type 1 diabetes a month later; the virus triggered my own immune cells to attack and render my pancreatic beta cells incapable of making any more insulin. If you have prediabetes or type 2 diabetes, though, the answer may be considerably less clear.

Regardless of how you got it, it's time to stop making excuses for not taking control of and conquering your own diabetes or prediabetes. In the rest of this chapter, you will not only learn about the first step you must take to achieve diabetes fitness, you will gain a better understanding of the basics you need to know to get started, including the reasons why becoming physically fit is the best and easiest way to effectively control your diabetes, how your body responds to physical activity, why being sedentary is so damaging to your body, and how to exercise safely with diabetes.

Are you genetically doomed to get diabetes?

Maybe both of your grandparents on one side of your family had type 2 diabetes and you've decided that you were genetically doomed from the start. Having immediate family members with type 2 diabetes certainly increases your risk of getting it yourself, but it's by no means a foregone conclusion. If you are a member of certain ethnic groups (African American, Hispanic or Latino, or Native American), your risk is higher to start with as well, but your ethnicity still doesn't doom you to getting it. Being overweight or obese and carrying that excess fat in your abdominal region also increases your risk, particularly if it's stored as **visceral fat** and not just directly under your skin, but as you now know, excess body fat is not as definitive a direct cause as was once believed. Okay, so maybe now you're down to blaming the food companies for creating too much tasty but unhealthy food and the TV producers for making their shows too interesting. Well, you may have a point . . . but let's look a little further anyway.

You can't blame it all on your genes

As much as you may want to, you should not simply blame the state of your health on your "bad" genes or some other uncontrollable factor; nor should you resign yourself to having poor BG control for the same reason. By way of example, take the Pima Native Americans of Arizona, who have an extremely high incidence of obesity, insulin resistance (prediabetes), and type 2 diabetes. In fact, since more than half of all Pima adults thirty-five years and older develop type 2 diabetes, researchers had previously concluded that if you were Native American, you were genetically doomed. Recently, another group of Pimas, from whom the Arizona group apparently descended, was discovered in Mexico. And interestingly enough, despite sharing the same gene pool, these two groups differ dramatically in their levels of body fat. The explanation? The Mexican Pimas are physically active farmers who eat a traditional diet of natural foods such as wheat, squash, beans, cactus buds, squawfish, and jackrabbit, while the Arizona Pimas eat highly refined, nutrient-poor foods and have adopted a sedentary lifestyle. And it's the Arizona Pimas who have type 2 diabetes.

Why all the concern about being unfit?

Currently, physical inactivity and a poor diet are together poised to overtake smoking as the leading cause of preventable death in the United States. Did you catch the key word in that sentence? Preventable. Even if it's only for the sake of prolonging your life, becoming physically fit is more than worth it—but there are numerous other reasons why it pays to become more physically active. For starters, it can reduce your risk of certain cancers (e.g., colon, prostate, and breast), help lower your blood pressure, prevent or reverse heart disease, reduce **depression** and anxiety, prevent thinning bones (**osteoporosis**), reverse prediabetes, and greatly lower your risk of developing diabetes. If you already have diabetes, being active can make good diabetes control a great deal more attainable.

The more sedentary you are, the greater your risk of dying prematurely from myriad causes becomes. Even more important, though, is your increased chance of not feeling good while you are alive. Honestly, would you really like to spend the last twenty years of your diabetes-shortened life impaired by **diabetic complications**? Why risk lowering your quality of life with diabetes when you can prevent it—and other chronic health problems—simply by becoming physically fit?

The real causes of unfitness today

Nearly half of all American adults report that they are not active at all, while 70 percent aren't moderately active enough to meet the recommended thirty minutes a day "most days of the week." Why are we all so sedentary? Blame it on the industrial revolution, and you won't be far off the mark. We're the modern-day "hunter-gatherers" who no longer do either. Moreover, in the past half century, Americans have experienced a rise in sedentary, leisure-time pursuits unparalleled in human history.

Labor-saving devices like dishwashers, remote controls, and personal computers have left most of us sitting on our (ever-expanding) derrieres more than ever. When was the last time you shopped on the Internet instead of walking in the mall? If your answer is "today," you are not alone. Not only do most American homes have at least one TV, but most also have one or more computers—usually with Internet access. In this fast-paced world of ours, is it any wonder that we often choose to let our fingers do the walking (on the keyboard) instead of our legs? And who twenty years ago could ever have imagined playing an Internet-linked video game on your cell phone? As a result of all these "improvements" to our way of life, we have become a society of unfit and fat people.

Of course, diet also plays a dramatic role in the current unfit state of most Americans. Not only have portion sizes increased during the past several decades, but we have also become entrenched in a "fast-food" mentality, leading us to expect and demand an ever greater selection of fast-food restaurants and low-nutrition, prepackaged food ready for consumption in supersized, "bargain" portions. And all this despite decreasing our energy needs with sedentary behaviors! We all tend to move around less after we gain excess weight from poor food choices, and the ensuing inactivity then causes us to gain more weight and become even less physically active—creating a vicious cycle. So, despite the proven and publicized health benefits of physical activity, the vast majority of us remain sedentary, unfit, and overweight.

We're even fatter than we think

Only a seemingly lucky minority of the American population is thin these days. Nearly a third of adults are obese, and more than two-thirds are overweight, leaving only a minority—one in three—anywhere near to supposedly "ideal" body weights. Without major, sweeping **lifestyle changes**, though, it appears unlikely that this obesity epidemic will be curtailed anytime soon. In fact, it appears that we're simply getting used to rising numbers of people with excess body fat.

As a nation, we're also being tricked into thinking that we're thinner than we really are. For example, did you know that clothing manufacturers secretly changed their sizes in the past decade by making a woman's dress size 10 today the equivalent of size 14 from a few decades ago? New sports stadiums are being constructed with wider seats, and Nike resized its size "small" sports bra to fit a bust that is two inches larger.

What really happens to the "couch potatoes"

The best way to avoid excess weight gain in the first place is to exercise regularly. A new study just concluded that America's youth are getting fat mainly because they don't move around enough, and the same is true for adults. As for the physiology of inactivity, a great deal of scientific evidence links a lack of physical activity directly to defects in the action of insulin at the level of your cells (primarily muscle and fat cells). Inside the muscle cells themselves, the ability to utilize oxygen declines with inactivity, resulting in a lower capacity for **aerobic** exercise and a reduction in your overall fitness—which in turn makes you feel less like exercising.

Although a lot of sitting around for any reason is unhealthy, TV watching appears to be especially detrimental, because your rate of energy expenditure (**metabolic** rate) is even lower while watching TV than while engaging in other sedentary activities, such as playing board games or even reading. Many pediatricians are now recommending that children be restricted from spending more than one to two hours a day using TVs and computers combined. Kids who watch a lot of TV are also more likely to have bad eating habits, such as munching on unhealthy, high-calorie snacks while watching the many junk food commercials targeting youth. The negative effects of excess TV time apparently last through adulthood as well, because the amount of time you spent watching TV during your childhood and adolescence is also directly associated with your risk of high **cholesterol**, diabetes, poor fitness, smoking, and obesity as an adult.

What does it mean to be "fit"?

When you see people who are overweight (even if you're one of them), do you automatically assume that they can't possibly be physically fit even if they exercise regularly? If so, it may be your definition of "fit" that needs to be revised. It's entirely possible to be fit even while carrying excess body fat. Actually, you may be way off base if you assume that a thin person is healthier than someone with more body fat. The latest research has shown that, while it's still best for your overall health to be fit and thin, being fit and fat is at least equal to being a thin, physically inactive "couch potato"—if not better.

Does becoming "fit" require a daily trip to the gym or engaging in physical activities you abhor? Luckily, the answer is no—or even fewer of us would ever achieve a fit state. It doesn't mean you have to be able to complete a marathon or a triathlon, but it does assume that you have the capacity to physically accomplish whatever you want to do without becoming unduly fatigued—such as walking up a flight of stairs; picking up your kids or grandkids; being on-the-go all day working, running errands, volunteering, or doing other activities without stopping much to rest; sleeping well at night and getting up the next day to do it all over again.

Being fit also implies that your body is healthy by current medical standards, which includes having a normal blood pressure, high levels of the good type of cholesterol (**HDL**) in your blood with low levels of the bad (**LDL**), very few risk factors for **cardiovascular disease** (the leading cause of death for all adults), and no major health problems. Fitness also implies high mental functioning and good emotional health, both of which can be negatively affected by the onset of many chronic health problems.

Of course, by the preceding definition of fitness, having diabetes would automatically disqualify you. However, a long and healthy life with diabetes is entirely achievable—assuming that you are willing to become more physically active and to take a long, hard look at your current diet. For instance, 16 weeks (or less) of 90 minutes of weekly vigorous exercise alone, without any weight loss, will vastly improve the action of your insulin as well as your fitness level—even if you are a middle-aged, overweight, sedentary, prediabetic man. If you restrict your calorie intake at the same time, you'll experience even greater improvements in your insulin action—maybe even enough to counterbalance any potential negative effects of having diabetes.

How important is your health to you, really?

What are you really willing to do to be healthy? If you were to develop a serious health problem—for example, heart disease, an ailment people with diabetes have a much higher risk of developing than people without diabetes—and your doctor were to tell you that taking a single "miracle" pill every day would cure you, you wouldn't forget to take it, would you? There's a reason why people always say, "If you don't have your health, you don't have anything." After all, who doesn't want to have good health? But Americans take more prescribed medicines than anyone else in the world, and many of us are still unhealthy.

So, what if the instructions from your doctor were instead to "take" that pill every day, put it in your pocket, and go out for a walk or a bike ride, to the park, to the gym, or anywhere to do anything physically active for at least 30 minutes a day? Does it still seem like a miraculous cure to you now? Given that more than half of people drop out of exercise programs within the first six months, in all likelihood the pill would be nothing more than a dud.

Exercise really is the best medicine

In my professional opinion, exercise truly is a "magic bullet" for optimizing quality of life, and if you have diabetes, the physical and mental health benefits are magnified. I'll recap some of the countless benefits for you. From a metabolic standpoint, it's always better to be fit, no matter your body weight. Exercise enhances your body's sensitivity to insulin, which usually results in better BG control; many chronic diseases in addition to type 2 diabetes are related to **insulin sensitivity** (including **hypertension** and heart disease). Exercise may also enhance your insulin production as long as enough beta cells remain in your pancreas. Regular exercise also lowers your risk of premature death, heart disease, certain types of cancers (colon, for example), anxiety and depression, osteoporosis, and severe arthritic symptoms. It even helps you sleep better, which is especially important since sleeping too little (e.g., only five hours a night) has been linked in recent studies with increased incidence of overweight and obesity, not to mention insulin resistance—even in healthy young adults. In fact, if exercise is not a potential cure for everything that ails you, then I really don't know what is.

Can you really prevent diabetes just by walking?

Type 2 diabetes may actually be preventable with regular physical activity—even just walking. During the past decade, many studies that assessed people's exercise habits have concluded that regular physical activity is associated with a lower risk for the development of type 2 diabetes. However, much of this research involved observational studies of large numbers of people using activity questionnaires or brief physical exams to assess their health status, lifestyle habits, and risk, and they relied heavily on often unreliable, self-reported exercise habits. Despite the fact that people tend to exaggerate their exercise habits, self-reported "active" individuals were still generally leaner than their sedentary counterparts, with lower levels of abdominal fat, better BG levels and insulin action, and a lower risk of developing diabetes.

More recently, landmark clinical trials have directly assessed the impact of regular physical activity on the prevention of type 2 diabetes. The Diabetes Prevention Program (DPP) studied 3,234 overweight American adults with **impaired glucose tolerance** (IGT, diagnosed with an oral **glucose** tolerance test) at high risk for diabetes, almost half of whom were from high-risk ethnicities (African Americans or Hispanics). Participants in the "lifestyle arm" of the study were asked to follow a low-fat diet and increase their exercise to include 150 minutes (2.5 hours) per week of a moderately intense activity (such as brisk walking) spread out over at least three days and engaged in for a minimum of 10 minutes at a time.

The news from this trial was so good that the study was actually wrapped up early. After just three years, people who had changed their lifestyles for the better had reduced their average risk of developing diabetes by a colossal 58 percent—despite their high-risk status. Moreover, this reduced risk was not dependent on ethnicity, age, or sex; in fact, the effect was even greater among older individuals. Moreover, a similar lifestyle study conducted in Finland studying high-risk individuals also resulted in exactly a 58 percent decrease in diabetes risk.

While the DPP study did not test the contribution of physical activity without simultaneous changes in diet and body weight, the active participants lost an average of only 7 percent of their body weight, equivalent to just 14 pounds in a 200-pound person or 21 pounds in a 300-pound person. Subjects in the Finnish study also lost body weight, ate less **saturated fat** and more **fiber**, and added 30 minutes of daily walking and occasional **resistance training** to their regimens. The study proved, among other things, the power of walking: subjects who walked 2.5 hours or more a week had a 63 to 69 percent lower risk of developing diabetes. It also found, however, that a person's genetic makeup can exert some influence over how effective lifestyle changes are in the prevention of diabetes. For some, total physical activity and a concomitant 5 to 7 percent weight loss had the greatest effect, while for others, the dietary changes appeared to result in a greater benefit.

Even if the protective effect of exercise on your risk for diabetes does vary somewhat depending on your genetic background, it's still a crucial addition to your lifestyle if you already have diabetes—for all of the physical health reasons discussed, and for some mental health ones that we will cover later (in fitness step 5).

It has now been proven that exercise alone can largely control or essentially reverse type 2 diabetes, and any exercise can help your insulin work better, regardless of what type you have. So why aren't people convinced of the importance of exercise? As with most things, maybe it's just that people need to be repeatedly hit over the head with a new idea before it finally sinks in.

But what if you already have diabetes?

There's another, equally important, reason for getting up off the couch if you already have diabetes, and that is that regular exercise is the key to good control of BG levels. The glucose-lowering effects of exercise can mainly be ascribed to a heightened sensitivity to insulin in exercised muscle, an effect that persists for only a day or two following the activity. This means that in order to maximize exercise's positive effects on BG control, you have to exercise regularly. Daily or near-daily activities are recommended; any type of exercise makes insulin work better. When your body needs less insulin, your pancreas is more likely to be able to produce enough to meet your body's needs, and your BG control will improve.

If you already have diabetes, any training-induced improvements are likely to be even more pronounced, and you can enjoy improvements in your diabetic control without significant weight loss. By way of example, a recent study of Japanese men and women with either prediabetes or type 2 diabetes (but who took no medications) reported that physical fitness by itself is equally important in staving off metabolic derangements. In that study, people who were classified as "low fit"—regardless of the amount of abdominal fat they had—had the greatest risk factors for heart disease. Those who were "moderate fit" or "high fit," though, had lower levels of insulin resistance, and the more fit they were, the better their fasting BG, insulin, and cholesterol levels, and their blood pressure readings.

Similarly, researchers in Finland found that if you have type 2 diabetes but engage in moderate or high levels of physical activity, you will be far less likely to die from heart disease than if you engage in only a low level of physical activity, regardless of your body mass, blood pressure, cholesterol levels, smoking status, or sex. People in the Finnish study who were moderately active (which included being active during work, during their commute to and from work, or during leisure time) reduced their risk of dying from heart disease by 39 percent, while highly active individuals had a 48 percent lower chance.

What walking by itself can do for your diabetes control

To prove the exact contribution of walking by itself, another recent study, the Diabetes In Control 10,000 step study, asked people with type 2 diabetes to increase their physical activity without changing their diets at all. Participants had to commit to taking at least 10,000 steps each day (equal to roughly 5 miles of walking), monitored with **pedometers**. A total of 44 diabetic adults completed the study, clocking in over 3 million steps, the equivalent of almost 15,000 collective miles over three months. For the diabetic adults in the study, many improvements occurred after just the first four weeks of the study. By the end of three months, over 15 participants had reduced their dosages of various medications (including diabetes-related medications), six had completely eliminated some medications, and three had gone off all medications completely, with no change in their diets and an average weight loss of only 4 measly pounds. The conclusion: if you wear a pedometer with a goal of becoming more active all day (increasing, say, from 3,000 steps to 10,000), you can improve your physical fitness level, BG level, cholesterol levels, blood pressure, and body weight.

Exercise can also prevent diabetic complications

Exercise may also play a role in preventing any potential complications related to poor glycemic control. Many diabetes-related complications (such as loss of sensation in the feet, eye disease, kidney problems, or heart disease) are related to having diabetes for a number of years, so the earlier it is diagnosed, the better your possible outcome. As you now know, diabetes is an extremely strong risk factor for heart disease, and physical inactivity increases your risk of dying from heart disease. With regular exercise, you can improve BG levels and reduce both contributors to heart disease risk at once.

Regular aerobic exercise also lessens the potential impact of most of the other cardiovascular risk factors, including elevated blood **lipids** (cholesterol and other blood fats), insulin resistance, obesity, and hypertension. High blood pressure is associated with higher levels of insulin, and regular physical activity can result in lower blood pressure and reduced circulating levels of insulin. If you have elevated blood pressure, though, it is best to avoid certain high-intensity or resistance exercises, which may cause blood pressure to rise dangerously high. Such activities include heavy weight training; near-maximal exercise of any type; activities that require intense, sustained contractions of the upper body—water skiing or wind surfing, for example; or exercises for which you must hold your breath.

Having diabetes, you also have a higher risk of joint-related injuries, so a moderate program of walking may be more suitable for you than a more vigorous activity such as running. Even walking on a regular basis can help you live longer. In fact, if you're a diabetic adult of any age and walk at least two hours per week, you'll have a 39 percent lower risk of dying from any cause and will reduce your risk of dying from heart disease by 34 percent. Some of my own research on older people with type 2 diabetes has shown that the skin circulation in their feet—where they are at risk for developing ulcers—is slightly improved right after exercise and from regular aerobic exercise training. Good BG control, then, when achieved with the help of regular physical activity, has the potential to prevent or delay almost all of the potential long-term health complications of diabetes.

Exercise and glucose-raising "stress" hormones

To better understand how exercise is likely to affect your BG levels, you need to know how your body handles physical activity. When you start to exercise, your body immediately responds by releasing **stress hormones** that work to increase your BG. At any given time, you have a relatively limited supply of glucose stored in your muscles and liver (i.e., **glycogen**) and far less circulating in your bloodstream, but your BG levels must be maintained for your brain and nervous system to function properly. Since **carbohydrates** are the primary fuel your body uses during any exercise, your liver must act quickly to replace the BG muscles use by breaking down its glycogen to form glucose or by making new glucose from lactic acid or other precursors.

The stress hormones released during exercise signal the liver to begin releasing more glucose. A pancreatic hormone called **glucagon** is the one with the most direct effect on that organ. Epinephrine (**adrenaline**) raises your heart rate and signals your exercising muscles to break down their stored glycogen—and some fat as well. At the same time, your body reduces the amount of insulin the pancreas is secreting, which helps to keep your muscles from taking up too much of the circulating glucose. Other hormones, such as norepinephrine, growth hormone, and **cortisol**, effectively redistribute more blood and provide other fuels to working muscles and the liver during physical activity.

While stress hormones are generally effective in maintaining BG levels during exercise, there may be times when your BG level is already higher than normal, such as after eating a meal loaded with rapidly absorbed carbohydrates. In this instance, you would like exercise to lower your BG level, not simply maintain it. However, exercise can raise, maintain, or lower BG levels: how fast you move, how hard you work out, and how long you are active can all affect the energy needs of your working muscles and can have various influences on your BG as well. For example, many endurance athletes develop **hypoglycemia** (low BG) at the end of a marathon-length run or workout due to the extreme demands that extended, high-intensity activities put on their bodies' carbohydrate stores. On the other hand, heavy weight lifting (involving hard bursts of activity done for only a short time) can actually cause your stress hormones to produce more BG than your body needs, causing BG levels to rise temporarily.

Which energy system your body uses—when and why

The best way, then, to anticipate your body's BG response to exercise is to understand which of your three energy systems predominates for your chosen activity. Regardless of the system used to supply energy, all muscular contractions are fueled directly by a substance known as **ATP (adenosine triphosphate)**. For short, powerful, **anaerobic** activities such as sprinting or heavy weight lifting, the first energy system, the **phosphagens** (stored ATP and creatine phosphate), makes ATP rapidly available to your muscles; however, this system will provide energy for only up to 10 seconds of all-out activity. Once it begins to lose its ATP-making capacity, the **lactic acid system**, your second system, gears up and provides additional energy for up to about two minutes total. Neither one of these systems uses oxygen (making them "anaerobic" by definition), but both make relatively little ATP so that their use actually slightly raises BG levels temporarily, due to the heightened release of stress hormones that accompanies them.

Your third and final energy system, the aerobic or **oxygen system**, fuels all activities that use the major muscle groups and are sustained for two minutes or longer by making large quantities of ATP oxidatively (by using oxygen), but at a slower rate than the first two systems. Your muscles must have access to a steady supply of ATP during prolonged activities such as walking, running, cycling, and swimming. The fuels supplying this system are any of the macronutrients stored in various depots around your body—carbohydrates in muscles, liver, and blood; fats in **adipose** and muscle; and **proteins** in muscle—making it the most versatile of the three energy systems.

When you are resting, your body usually uses a mix of about 60 percent fat and 40 percent carbohydrate (with insignificant protein use), but during exercise, carbohydrates supply the majority of the fuel—even more so when you work out harder. Depletion of both your muscle glycogen and BG is inevitable if the activity is prolonged. Your body can also use fat, but fat contributes most during mild- to moderate-intensity workouts. During recovery from exercise, though, when your body is restocking depleted fuels, fat use predominates.

Intense exercise affects your BG control differently

Why would anyone choose to exercise intensely if it raises BG levels? One reason is that the effect is temporary: your BG will usually return to normal within an hour or two afterward. More relevant is the fact that almost any exercise may enhance your insulin sensitivity and glucose tolerance for a period of time afterward, making physical activity of utmost importance to diabetes prevention and control. Both recent exercise and regular exercise training appear to have favorable effects on BG levels and insulin action in almost everyone. For starters, when carbohydrate use is significant, as it is during 30 minutes of continuous moderate exercise, your BG levels decrease during the activity. Then, for two or more hours afterward, prior activity causes your muscles to take up more BG with very little insulin. In fact, a single workout—particularly if prolonged or intense—can enhance your insulin action for 24 hours or more while your glycogen stores in muscles and liver are being replenished.

In addition, high-intensity workouts such as repeated **interval training** result in significant depletion of your muscle glycogen, thereby increasing your risk for later-onset hypoglycemia, particularly if you take certain **oral diabetic medications** or insulin (more on these in step 6). To prevent this, you may need to consume moderate amounts of carbohydrate within 30 minutes of exhaustive, glycogen-depleting exercise to allow your muscles to more rapidly restore the glycogen you used up.

Good control of your BG levels during this period is essential, though; if your diabetes is poorly controlled after your exercise session, you're likely to experience reduced rates of muscle glycogen repletion. Thus, to maintain glycemic control, you may still need to take some additional insulin (if you use it) to cover your carbohydrate intake.

Is exercising in the morning different than exercising in the afternoon?

Another variable that you may have to factor in is the time of day you do your physical activities. Many people experience a transient state of insulin resistance first thing in the morning that is attributable to the increase in hormones that help maintain BG when you go overnight without eating; the two with the biggest anti-insulin effect in the morning are cortisol and growth hormone.

A recent study showed that in moderately hyperglycemic type 2 diabetic men treated with oral diabetic medications, one hour of moderate cycling caused their BG levels to decrease minimally when they exercised before eating breakfast, but drop dramatically (down to almost normal) when exercising two hours after eating breakfast. Thus, it is best to eat (and take your diabetic medications) before exercising in the early morning if you want to have the greatest effect on your BG level. On the other hand, if you tend to drop too low during activities, then exercising at that time of day may be your best bet to preventing hypoglycemia from occurring at all.

Any training makes your insulin work better

If you're physically trained, you will generally have a heightened sensitivity to insulin—but why? It appears that the answer varies according to the type of training you do. For instance, in lean but sedentary young adult women (ages eighteen to thirty-five) engaging in six months of thrice weekly either endurance (aerobic) or resistance (weight) training, both forms of training improved their glucose use, but by different mechanisms. Weight training apparently results in enhancements in your muscle mass, allowing for greater overall glucose uptake. While endurance training does not increase your muscle mass as much, it does enhance your muscular uptake of BG without changes in body weight or abdominal fat.

What if you're older or overweight? Training will still work for you. Sedentary, insulin-resistant, middle-aged adults engaging in 30 minutes of moderate walking three to seven days per week for six months succeeded in reversing their prediabetic state—without changing their diets or losing any body weight. In older adults (average of 72 years), all it took was low- to moderate-intensity "walking" on mini-trampolines for 20 to 40 minutes four days per week over a four-month period to enhance their glucose uptake without any additional insulin release or loss of abdominal fat.

If you're young but obese, you're still in luck. Studies have shown that, regardless of your age, exercise training can improve your insulin action within just one week of training without weight loss or a true training adaptation in muscle.

TIP

1

NO MATTER YOUR WEIGHT

NO MATTER your weight or age, physical activity can improve your insulin action, reverse prediabetes, prevent type 2 diabetes, and control your BG. Just 30 minutes a day of moderate walking three to seven days a week may be all it takes—even if you don't change your diet or lose any weight. Even a single week of training will improve your insulin action. Add in resistance training for additional benefits and extra gains in muscle mass.

Add in some weights to really power up your insulin

In addition to walking, you might want to do some weight training as well to further improve your sensitivity to insulin and better control your BG levels. In people with type 2 diabetes, four to six weeks of moderate-intensity (40 to 50 percent of maximal) resistance training improved their insulin sensitivity by 48 percent without causing any significant changes in their body fat or muscle mass. Similarly, newly diagnosed type 2 diabetic men who did 16 weeks of "progressive" resistance training (the resistance lifted was increased over time) just twice a week gained muscle mass, lost body fat (particularly in the abdominal region), and greatly enhanced their insulin action—all despite a 15 percent increase in the amount of calories they consumed. Likewise, if you're an older, type 2 diabetic woman, the combination of aerobic and resistance training may afford even greater improvements in your insulin action and a more significant decrease in your abdominal fat than aerobic training alone, with increased muscle mass to boot.

Why "diet" truly is a four-letter word

Not everyone likes to exercise. I know that just telling you that you need to do it is not necessarily going to work. Maybe you're the kind of person who'd rather go on a diet than have to lift anything heavier than your fork. Let me put a question to you then: since millions of Americans are currently dieting and countless others have already been on one or more diets, why isn't everyone thin?

How many times have you yourself lost 10, 20, or even 30 or more pounds, only to gain it all back over time? The problem isn't that you can't lose weight on a diet—usually you can, as long as you eat fewer calories than your body needs. Even with diabetes, you can lose weight on the famed Atkins "low-carb" diet, mostly because cutting all of the carbohydrates out of your diet causes you to consume significantly fewer calories. The real problem is not losing weight while on the diet; it's keeping the weight off. Even among successful dieters, an estimated 95 percent regain the same amount (or more) within six months to a year.

Since you may find yourself, postdiet, eating the same kinds of foods you ate pre-diet, the typical rebound response is an excessive intake of calories—particularly in the form of extra fat. Thus you lose the battle against returning to your previous, higher "set" body weight. While this set point can change gradually over your lifetime, it remains the same over the relatively short time-frame of a diet. Therefore, if you don't adopt permanent lifestyle changes that allow you to gradually reset your body weight to a new, lower one, you will be doomed to regain your lost weight. Also, rapid or extreme weight loss invariably results in a loss of body water and muscle—the loss of which adds to the ease of regaining weight once you resume your normal food intake.

If you have to choose between dieting (and likely regaining all the weight in the end) and becoming more fit, choose the latter. When you experience large fluctuations in body weight over time (also known as "yo-yo" dieting because your weight goes up and down, up and down), you're likely to be less healthy than people who never lost any or lost very little of their excess body fat. Women whose body weight cycles in this manner may actually have a much greater risk of developing heart disease.

TIP
2

────────── **NO MATTER YOUR WEIGHT** ──────────

THE REALITY of dieting is that, over the long haul, it just does not work for most people. Not only does it become progressively harder to lose weight the longer you stay on a diet (thus making it harder for you to stay motivated to follow it), but at least nine out of ten dieters who have successfully lost weight ultimately regain the pounds that they struggled to shed. In fact, most people gain back even more weight than they originally lost, regardless of the diet they followed.

If you did lose weight, you don't have to gain it back

Okay, so a few lucky people take the weight off and keep it off, and maybe you're one of them. If so, congratulations are in order. It takes a special person to keep the weight off. Interested in knowing what sets apart those people who are successful in losing a lot of weight by dieting and not regaining it? Over the past decade, the National Weight Control Registry has tracked individuals who have lost at least 30 pounds and kept the weight off for at least a year. Although that may not sound very hard, keeping lost weight off for a year is actually quite uncommon even among successful dieters, since you're most likely to regain the weight you lost within the first six months after the diet ends.

Their results confirm what we **exercise physiologists** have known all along: exercise matters. It doesn't appear to make any difference what method or weight loss plan the successful dieters used to lose weight (they used everything from a conventional lower-calorie, moderate-carbohydrate diet like Weight Watchers to the famed "low-carb" Atkins one). What matters are the two lifestyle habits that almost all of them adopt to keep their weight down. That is, they continue to be conscientious about what they eat (more healthful food in appropriate portions), and they exercise almost daily, expending about 2,000 calories a week in physical activity. So, if you want to maintain your weight loss, get up off the couch and go for a walk (and do it again tomorrow, and the next day, and the next).

But what about 10 or 20 years down the road?

You may be able to keep your weight down for a year or two, but what about 10 or 20 years from now? In reality, most Americans have very little success in preventing the weight gain that comes with aging. Does this mean that if you are of a certain age you should give up trying to prevent gaining any more weight or that you are undeniably doomed to suffer from being overweight and out of shape? Absolutely not! The solution is simply to get active and to stop worrying so much about maintaining a specific weight.

Exactly why is expending extra energy through exercise so important? Surprisingly, despite the hundreds of thousands of calories—even millions for some—that you eat in the course of a year, your body is capable of maintaining its weight within a pound or two—which demonstrates the innate aptitude of the human body to tightly match food intake with calorie use. The fact that more people than ever before are gradually becoming overweight despite this inborn ability to auto-regulate our body weight is primarily the result of expending too few calories through physical activity.

Excess weight often "creeps" on, which means that it comes on slowly and steadily over a number of years, a little bit at a time. It also means that it's never too late for you to prevent or reverse this trend with small changes in your daily habits. For instance, if you eat just 50 calories a day more than you use (equal to only a small apple or about two Hershey's chocolate kisses), your total weight gain from that excess alone will be 5 pounds of body fat a year, given that a pound of fat equals approximately 3,500 calories. Similarly, if you have an excess intake of closer to 100 calories daily, you'll gain 10 pounds in a year. If, however, you take in 50 calories less a day (by leaving a few bites uneaten at each meal or skipping a small treat) and then expend an extra 50 calories a day—easily accomplished with some extra walking, stretching, or other mild activity—you can lose 10 pounds of body fat in a year instead. Which would you rather do?

TIP

3

NO MATTER YOUR WEIGHT

THOSE SUCCESSFUL dieters who do not regain the weight they lost while dieting have a few key behaviors in common. Almost all of them continue to watch what they eat after they stop officially dieting; exercise regularly for close to 60 minutes a day (mainly walking); and eat a healthy breakfast every day.

A doctor's "prescription" to lose weight may do more harm than good

When you found out about your diabetes from your doctor, he or she probably told you to lose weight, eat better, take your medications, and exercise more. Maybe the recommendations were not laid out in exactly that order, but I would bet that weight loss was one of the top recommendations. However, since long-term dieting has such a high failure rate, a blanket prescription for heavier people to lose weight has the potential to harm you more than help you. Although some weight loss may improve your insulin sensitivity, losing large amounts of weight will likely be unnecessary—not to mention unrealistic—to achieve your BG goal. Thus—and I can't stress this enough—your success at controlling your BG should not be pinned on significant weight loss or some unattainable target body weight.

Consider the case of one woman diagnosed with diabetes in her early forties. At the time she weighed 270 pounds, which categorized her as "morbidly obese," and her glycated hemoglobin, which should have been 7 percent or lower to be well controlled, was almost double that at 14 percent. Over the next few months, she started eating better and exercising more, and her overall diabetes control vastly improved: her glycated hemoglobin levels dropped to 8 percent and then to under 6 percent—reflective of an average BG level within normal, nondiabetic limits—over that period of time. When she saw her doctor again, he expressed disappointment about her progress solely because she had not lost any weight. In fact, he told her in no uncertain terms that she obviously didn't care about her health since weight loss should be her main focus and she was failing to lose any.

Not only was this physician's fixation on weight loss misguided (since he ignored the vast improvements in her diabetes management accomplished without weight loss), it was also emotionally counterproductive for the woman, failing to give her the encouragement and praise she deserved for so effectively managing her BG levels on her own. As an exercise physiologist, I can tell you that embarking on a new program of regular exercise can actually make you gain weight rather than lose it in the short term. This most likely just means that your body composition is changing for the better—that you are gaining muscle while losing body fat. In my opinion, physicians would serve patients far better by monitoring short-term changes in their body-fat levels instead of their scale weight.

TIP
4

_____ **NO MATTER YOUR WEIGHT** _____

FORGET STRICT dieting, fad eating plans, or obsessing over what you are eating because of your weight. Even with small reductions in your weight (such as 5 to 7 percent, or no more than 10 to 15 pounds for most people), which often occur over time as you become more active and make small changes in your dietary patterns, the majority of health benefits can and will be yours. Lifestyle choices play the biggest role in determining whether you develop obesity, prediabetes, or diabetes, and these conditions can all be improved without dieting.

Why exercise makes your body weight change more slowly

About the only thing that exercise can't do is make your body weight go down faster than dieting alone—if you have decided to go on a diet. This phenomenon is not inherently bad, and it deserves a fuller explanation.

When you diet, the weight that you lose is a combination of body fat, muscle mass, and water weight. By exercising, you actually help retain and even gain some muscle mass, which is good since muscle is sensitive to the effects of insulin and is a good place to store your extra glucose. The downside of retaining or gaining muscle—if it really can be considered a downside—is that muscle is denser than body fat and, thus, it weighs more. Consequently, you can lose fat while retaining or gaining muscle with exercise, and your weight on the scales may change very little (or even rise slightly at first), even though your body composition is undeniably changing for the better.

TIP
5

_____ **NO MATTER YOUR WEIGHT** _____

DON'T LET your bathroom scale get you down. When you start exercising more, your weight may not go down very quickly, and it may even go up for a while—but such changes are far from meaning that you aren't making any headway. Muscle mass is more dense than body fat, so muscle weighs more. You can lose body fat while gaining muscle and actually gain weight. Pay more attention to your waist and hip measurements and to how loose your clothes are getting than to your weight on a regular scale. In fact, if you must weigh yourself, don't do it more than once a week, and always do it at the same time of day under similar circumstances (e.g., before eating breakfast).

Use exercise to stop gaining more weight

An added benefit of exercise is that even if it doesn't help you lose all of the weight you want to, it can still prevent you from gaining weight while you positively modify your body composition (that is, you lose fat while gaining muscle). Many adults are still trying to lose or maintain their body weight by dieting, yet very few are also using exercise. In my opinion, dieters must be avoiding exercise either out of ignorance or out of an unwillingness to believe how important it is to weight control.

Even though weight loss may be slower when exercise is part of the regimen, making lifestyle changes is a much better method of both accomplishing better BG control and losing weight than using supplemental insulin to improve overall diabetes control. When people with type 2 diabetes implement lifestyle changes (exercise and dietary modifications) alone, their diabetes control improves similarly to those who either have just begun using insulin or who implement the same lifestyle changes along with using insulin. However, if you are using supplemental insulin, you're likely to end up gaining as much or more weight over the course of a year than you'll lose by making lifestyle changes alone. Be forewarned, however, that you will lose almost all of the glycemic and body weight improvements if you fail to maintain your lifestyle changes.

Extra body fat unfairly gets too much of the blame

Is excess body fat really the only culprit in your diminishing insulin action, and do you really need to lose all of your excess fat to be healthy? The worldwide type 2 diabetes epidemic is unquestionably following closely on the heels of an increase in fatness around the world, and about 90 percent of newly diagnosed diabetic individuals are either overweight or obese. As a result, your extra fat gets blamed for everything from elevated cholesterol levels to heart disease. In addition to type 2 diabetes, researchers have held obesity directly responsible for **hyperinsulinemia** (elevated levels of the hormone insulin in the blood) and glucose intolerance (both indicative of prediabetes), congestive heart failure, gallstones, gout, arthritis, sleep apnea, some types of cancer (endometrial, breast, prostate, and colon), infertility and menstrual irregularities in women, and psychological disorders.

But the big question is whether the coexistence of such conditions with excess body fat actually proves that excess weight is the cause of them. Fat cells (a.k.a. "adipose cells," or "adipocytes") are still poorly understood, but we do know that they're far from dormant, as was previously believed. In truth, fat actually "talks" to other parts of your body by releasing hormones such as **leptin** and **adiponectin** that affect food intake, fat storage, and more. While the actions of other lesser-known, fat-derived hormones are not well understood, it is known that leptin may have direct effects on the liver's storage of glucose—which determines whether an obese person becomes diabetic. Excess body fat and some of these health problems are thus certainly linked, but exactly how has not yet been made clear.

Nonetheless, many scientists and clinicians are guilty of incorrectly claiming that the coexistence of obesity with conditions such as insulin resistance, hypertension, and type 2 diabetes irrefutably proves cause and effect—that excess body fat is the direct cause of these conditions—despite evidence to the contrary. For example, following endurance training, your fat cells become more responsive to insulin, as do your muscle cells, whether you lose weight or not—and both types of cells are thought to contribute heavily to insulin resistance. We can also look at the example of isolated fat cells taken from nondiabetic people: these fat cells can respond normally to insulin in a test tube even when they came from insulin-resistant donors. There has to be something more going on than excess fat alone if the same fat cells are insulin resistant in a person's body but not in a lab.

Blame your muscles, liver, or beta cells instead?

We need a new explanation. Let's look at what else might be going on in your body when excess weight is gained. Along with your adipose cells, both your muscles and your liver store extra fat as you gain weight. More fat storage in your muscles may decrease the uptake of BG into those areas, thus making them more resistant to the usual effects of insulin. This can have a tremendous impact, because your muscles are responsible for the majority of BG uptake and use in response to insulin. Paradoxically, though, regular exercisers actually store more fat in their muscles without experiencing insulin resistance—which would lead us to conclude that the amount of fat stored in muscles may not be critical.

On the other hand, the latest research indicates that storing extra fat in your liver may contribute to a state of low-level **inflammation** throughout your body and that this leads to the development of insulin resistance, diabetes, heart disease, and other metabolic disorders. The liver, therefore, may prove to be a crucial link between weight gain and the development of prediabetes and type 2 diabetes. But wait— unfortunately, it's not quite that clear-cut. One of the primary contributors to this systemic inflammation present in diabetes is believed to be an inflammatory compound called **TNF-alpha** (tumor necrosis factor-alpha), which can be produced by your adipose tissue as well as other tissues, such as muscles, bones, and the cells lining your blood vessels. So which tissue is really releasing the TNF-alpha that is making you insulin resistant? We don't know. Thankfully, we do know that regular exercise can inhibit the production of TNF-alpha and its resulting inflammation, thus potentially preventing or reversing insulin resistance. However, that still leaves us uncertain about the exact roles our muscles, fat cells, and liver (or possibly other body tissues) play in all of this.

Researchers have discovered, in mice at least, receptors on certain cells where **free fatty acids** (blood fats commonly elevated in overweight people) can bind and have a negative effect—and they're located not on muscle, fat, or liver cells, but rather on the pancreatic beta cells. The mice that lack these receptors (meaning that the effect of these free fatty acids does not come into play) do not gain excess body weight even when they eat extra calories. The existence of similar receptors—which would cause increased insulin release contributing to eventual beta cell failure and weight gain with excessive calorie and fat intake—in humans is also a distinct possibility, but one that remains to be studied.

The many faces of insulin resistance

It appears, therefore, that scientists may have jumped to the wrong conclusion when they decided to blame fat cells alone for everything that ails you. Granted, the vast majority of insulin-resistant people (with prediabetes or type 2 diabetes) are indeed overweight, but not all people who are overweight are insulin resistant. You can reverse prediabetes without a significant loss of body fat simply by implementing positive changes in your exercise and dietary habits. As shown in the following table, many factors besides weight loss can improve your body's insulin sensitivity and, consequently, reverse prediabetes or improve diabetes control.

Other Factors That Can Improve Insulin Sensitivity

- ▶ Regular aerobic and resistance exercise
- ▶ Muscle mass gain
- ▶ Loss of body fat—particularly intra-abdominal (visceral) fat, extra fat stored in the liver, and possibly some of the excess fat in muscles
- ▶ Improved BG control
- ▶ Reduced levels of circulating free fatty acids (one type of fat in blood)
- ▶ Reduction in low-level, systemic inflammation (via suppression of TNF-alpha)
- ▶ More effective action of leptin, causing reduced food intake
- ▶ Reduction in mental (anxiety, depression) and/or physical (illness, etc.) stressors
- ▶ Decrease in circulating levels of cortisol
- ▶ Increased testosterone levels in men
- ▶ Intake of more dietary fiber, less saturated and **trans fat**, and fewer highly refined foods
- ▶ Daily consumption of a healthy breakfast
- ▶ Lower caffeine intake
- ▶ Adequate sleep (seven to eight hours a night for most adults)
- ▶ Effective treatment of sleep apnea
- ▶ Use of insulin-sensitizing medications

Most health-care providers—myself included—have been guilty of counseling people about the health wonders of weight loss, with the (usually unattainable) goal being the permanent achievement of an ideal or nearly ideal body weight and shape. Unfortunately, most medical and health organizations are still on the bandwagon today, taking the position that if you don't lose a significant amount of weight, your health will suffer. While excess body fat is clearly not entirely harmless, it's safe to say that the purported health benefits of substantial weight loss have likely been greatly exaggerated.

TIP

6

NO MATTER YOUR WEIGHT

EXCESS BODY fat is more appropriately considered a symptom of associated health conditions such as diabetes or as one contributor to their development rather than as their sole cause. A sedentary lifestyle is likely a bigger contributor to insulin resistance and diabetes than body fat alone.

Does your body shape make a difference?

Where you store your excess body fat may be more important to your health than how much of it you have. Body fat patterning, unfortunately, is genetically predetermined, meaning that you can control only the total amount of fat that you store, not where your body puts it. Your patterning is reflected in your **waist-to-hip ratio** (**WHR**). Your waist is measured as the circumference (in inches or centimeters) at your belly button, while hip measures are taken around the widest part (wherever that may be) of your buttocks. Due to inherent anatomical differences between men and women, optimal WHR differs by sex. A WHR of less than or equal to 0.9 reduces metabolic risk for men, while 0.8 is the cutoff for women. For either sex, a WHR greater than 1.0 places you in the danger zone for undesirable health problems.

A high WHR, otherwise known as **abdominal obesity** (an apple body shape more typical in men), results from a greater amount of fat tissue being stored deep within the abdominal cavity, in and around the internal organs. This more metabolically active visceral fat is easier to gain and lose, but it's also commonly associated with metabolic disorders such as insulin resistance, type 2 diabetes, high blood pressure, and heart disease. Being heavier around the hips and thighs (pear-shaped) is more common in women and less associated with metabolic derangements. As far as your shape goes, it's far better to be a pear than an apple.

Using the WHR to assess diabetes risk may not be as effective as using just the **waist circumference** measurement. For men at least, the bigger their waist, the greater their risk of developing type 2 diabetes. Men with waists that are 37.9 to 39.8 inches in circumference, for example, have a risk of developing diabetes five times greater than men whose waists are 29 to 34 inches, likely due to increased visceral fat. Women's waists, though, should be less than 34.7 inches in circumference to lower diabetes risk.

TIP

7

NO MATTER YOUR WEIGHT

WE CAN no longer conclude that obesity and overweight invariably cause a state of insulin resistance, prediabetes, type 2 diabetes, or even heart disease, because many overweight people reverse these conditions with lifestyle changes alone. While being overly fat is certainly not devoid of health risks, weight loss—

specifically body fat loss—alone is apparently neither a panacea nor a strict requirement for becoming fit or living well.

Why you should exercise to change your shape for the better

If you have a large belly, don't give up all hope yet. At least you now know that impaired insulin action is more directly linked to how much visceral (intra-abdominal) fat you have than any other type of body fat. So why not just go on a diet instead of breaking a sweat exercising? A recent study looked at the effects of dieting, aerobic exercise, and a combination of the two in obese older women with type 2 diabetes in an attempt to definitively answer that question. After 14 weeks, the women's body weight and total body fat decreased the same amount whether they simply followed a low-calorie diet high in **monounsaturated fats** (like those found in many nuts, olive oil, and vegetables) or simultaneously dieted and exercised (moderate walking for 50 minutes three times a week). In the group that exercised without dieting, though, weight loss was minimal. That group's body fat did decrease some, but less than half as much as in the other two groups.

So far, you're probably not convinced that exercise is worth it, but just hold on—there's more. The researchers also measured both the amount of visceral fat lost as well as the less harmful **subcutaneous** (below your skin) variety, and here is where all of the exercisers clearly prevailed: only if you exercise—regardless of whether you lose any weight—will you lose any of your unhealthy visceral fat. Dieting by itself, while reducing your subcutaneous and total abdominal fat, does not appear to get rid of the visceral type. Moreover, if you exercise but don't diet, you'll keep all of your muscle mass, and if you exercise and diet, you'll still lose less muscle than if you diet only. Along the same lines, if you lose weight from dieting alone, you won't get rid of extra fat stored in muscle, but—you guessed it—if you exercise, you will. If you have to choose between exercise and dieting for better diabetes control and improved insulin sensitivity, choose exercise every time.

NO MATTER YOUR WEIGHT

ALTHOUGH BEING overly fat is not ideal for your health, any potentially negative metabolic effects of excess body fat can be favorably moderated to a large
extent by becoming fit and remaining regularly active.

Fit and fat is where it's at

Even if you can't lose all the weight you want to, you can achieve a
higher level of fitness, and doing so will undeniably benefit your health.
Over the years, researchers have examined the effects of being fat
and/or fit, separately and combined, on the risk of developing a debili-
tating illness or dying. The main finding has been that as your weight
increases, so does your risk of dying from heart disease or developing
diabetes. On a more positive note, the more physically fit you are, the
lower your risk of dying—from any cause—becomes. In other words, fat
weight gain and unfitness are independent risk factors for heart disease,
mortality, and diabetes. The best scenario is still to be "fit and thin," but
although becoming fit can't completely reverse your elevated risks if
you're overweight, being classified as "fit and fat" at least puts you
closer to people who are thin but unfit. The worst thing to be, indis-
putably, is a member of the "unfit and fat" club.

Why is being unfit so damaging to your body? The wonderful, insulin-
sensitizing effects of acute exercise and exercise training mentioned previously are transient, meaning that they don't last long after you revert to a
sedentary state. The effects of a single workout may last from one hour
(following short, mild exercise) up to a day or two (for prolonged, intense
activities), and the effects of regular training begin to reverse within just two
to three days. Granted, if you have increased your muscle mass with training, all of your health gains will not be lost in such a short period of time,
but with continued inactivity, they certainly will be. The saying "Use it or
lose it" definitely applies to training-induced changes in insulin action and
BG control, as well as to all of exercise's other health benefits.

TIP
9

NO MATTER YOUR WEIGHT

PHYSICAL ACTIVITY makes a huge difference in whether you will experience overall weight gain, maintenance, or loss, especially in the context of modern-day
access to excess calories and labor-saving devices. Even expending an extra 50
calories a day more than you take in can result in a weight loss of five pounds over
the course of a year.

Daily activity—plus a healthy diet—is the best practice

If you combine exercise with dietary changes, you may fare even better yet. Diabetic participants in Pritikin Longevity Center studies who
followed diets high in fiber and complex carbohydrates, but very low in
refined sugars, cholesterol, fat, and salt, and who engaged in 30 minutes or more of daily exercise, experienced remarkable results. Almost
75 percent of the people taking oral diabetic medications were able to
discontinue them, and close to 40 percent on insulin injections controlled their BG levels without any extra insulin—after just three weeks
of the program. Although they lost some weight, their postprogram
body fatness was far from ideal—yet their diabetes control was vastly
improved.

If you're a regular exerciser, a less healthy diet will likely not have a
negative impact on your insulin action. The relative glycemic effect of
foods will be lower because your insulin can function more effectively
to lower any glycemic spikes after eating. In other words, an overweight but fit individual uses carbohydrate better just by having more
insulin-responsive muscles. Not exercising is thus a potentially more
potent contributor to ineffective diabetes management than misguided
dietary choices. It also makes sense, however, that regular exercise
alone, without any attention paid to eating well, will have less of an influence on the prevention or control of diabetes than a combination of the
two lifestyle changes. For that reason, a quality diet is also an important
component in treating diabetes, and the two are best done together—
that is, daily activity plus a healthier diet.

As I mentioned previously, physical activity can have a huge effect on
the action of insulin, and ineffective insulin is a universal problem in
people with diabetes or prediabetes. Accordingly, the only time your

body can effectively handle a high intake of rapidly absorbed carbohydrate foods without concomitant spikes in your BG is when you exercise long and/or hard. In those cases, a significant amount of your muscle glycogen is used up, and consuming carbohydrates during the activity may be useful in providing glucose to delay fatigue, particularly when you exercise for longer than an hour. For a couple of hours following exercise, such carbohydrates can also be taken up from the bloodstream more easily—with very little insulin needed—to replenish depleted muscle glycogen stores. Eating carbohydrate foods high in fat (such as doughnuts) during exercise, though, would not be appropriate, since fat slows the absorption of carbohydrates.

Exercising safely and effectively with diabetes

With practice and a BG meter, you can manage your BG levels with any exercise regimen and gain all of the health benefits of regular exercise. Before you start, though, there are some potential risks of exercising with diabetes that you should be aware of in order to prevent and treat them effectively should they occur.

Blood glucose control. Fortunately, with regular training of any sort, your enhanced insulin sensitivity alone will invariably improve your BG control. While aerobic exercise generally has a moderate glucose-lowering effect, this can vary. As I mentioned, the type of exercise (easy, moderate, or intense) has a big effect on glycemic responses, and intense activities can temporarily raise BG levels. Prolonged activities, by using a mixture of fat, muscle glycogen, and blood glucose, seldom have that effect. Although mild activities like walking generally allow for more fat use, circulating glucose use can become quite significant as muscle glycogen stores become depleted, increasing your risk (albeit small) of developing low BG. Moreover, during higher-intensity, prolonged aerobic activities such as running (at greater than 65 percent of maximal capacity), your body relies exclusively on carbohydrates; depletion of both muscle glycogen and glucose in your bloodstream is inevitable if you exercise for longer than two hours. An intense activity such as repeated interval training results in significant depletion of muscle glycogen as well, thereby increasing your BG use for hours afterward—and your risk of later-onset hypoglycemia.

Your training status must also be considered when predicting your glycemic response to an activity. Becoming aerobically trained increases the proportion of fat your body uses for similar low- or moderate-intensity activity done after training. Using a greater proportion of fat spares muscle glycogen and blood glucose and allows you to more easily control your BG levels. Changes in your body's fuel use with training will, however, require you to make small adjustments to carbohydrate or insulin intake to maintain control over your BG levels.

Recognition and prevention of hypoglycemia. You can avoid developing hypoglycemia during or following physical activity with early recognition of its symptoms and rapid treatment. Hypoglycemia, usually defined as a BG level lower than 65 mg/dl (3.6 **mM**), requires immediate treatment when symptoms begin to occur; therefore, it is important to be able to recognize them. The following list should help.

Prevent hypoglycemia by keeping a BG meter handy to check your BG before, occasionally during (particularly for new, unusual, or extended activities), and after exercise. It can be useful to check immediately after exercise, and then every 30 to 60 minutes for a couple of hours to determine what kind of lasting effect the exercise is having on you. Eat rapidly absorbed carbohydrates as soon as your BG level begins to drop lower than you would like it to or any time you have symptoms of hypoglycemia (your BG meter might be wrong).

Common Symptoms of Hypoglycemia

- ► Cold or clammy skin
- ► Dizziness or lightheadedness
- ► Double or blurred vision
- ► Elevated pulse rate
- ► Headache
- ► Inability to do basic math
- ► Insomnia
- ► Irritability
- ► Mental confusion
- ► Nausea
- ► Nightmares
- ► Poor physical coordination
- ► Rapid-onset fatigue (sudden, unusual, or unexpected tiredness)
- ► Shakiness in your hands
- ► Sweating
- ► Tingling of hands or tongue

▶ Visual spots
▶ Weakness

If you're controlling your diabetes with diet and exercise alone, your risk of developing low BG during exercise is minimal—it's no higher than for someone without diabetes. For more intense activities of shorter duration, supplementing with a small amount of extra carbohydrates (5 to 10 grams) before you start can effectively prevent BG levels from dropping excessively. Prolonged exercise has a greater potential to make you hypoglycemic, both during and afterward. Eating a moderate amount (15 grams) of carbohydrate during and within 30 minutes of exhaustive, glycogen-depleting exercise will lower your risk of developing low BG levels and allow your body to more efficiently restore your preexercise levels of muscle glycogen.

Your risk of developing hypoglycemia is greater if you take certain diabetic medications that lower BG levels—primarily those that increase the secretion of insulin, such as Amaryl or Glucotrol (please refer to step 6)—or if you are taking insulin injections. To participate in more prolonged exercise training, you may need to consult with your healthcare provider about reducing doses of oral medications and/or insulin to prevent hypoglycemia.

If you are using insulin, you must be even more vigilant about anticipating and preventing hypoglycemia. When you are at rest, insulin alone facilitates the uptake of glucose into muscle and fat cells; during exercise, however, insulin levels would normally decrease since muscle contractions increase your glucose uptake directly without insulin. Because injected insulin can't be shut off as your pancreas would shut off its own supply of insulin, your cells will take up more glucose due to the combined uptake of glucose by muscle contractions and by this extra insulin. As a result, if you use insulin, you have a much greater risk of developing low BG during and after exercise. You may need to lower your insulin doses before and/or after long exercise sessions to prevent problems. For regular, planned exercise, you may be able to gauge how to effectively lower pre-exercise insulin doses on your own (by determining the glycemic effects of the activity) using the detailed, activity-specific guide for insulin users available in *The Diabetic Athlete*.

Treatment of hypoglycemia. Treat your low BG immediately with small amounts (5 to 10 grams) of readily absorbed carbohydrates, such as the ones listed in the following table. Wait 5 to 10 minutes for them to take effect, then recheck your glucose levels. Consume the same amount of carbohydrate again only if your hypoglycemic symptoms have not begun to resolve. Do not overtreat a low by eating too much (although the urge to do so is strong), or you'll end up battling high BG levels on the rebound.

High-carbohydrate sports bars like Power Bars are best used only to prevent, not to treat, low BG levels during activities (and should be consumed in quarters at a time to prevent overloading with carbohydrate). Whole fruits are not the best thing to eat because of their high fiber content (which slows the absorption of their carbohydrates) and high **fructose** (fruit sugar) content. Also, never attempt to treat hypoglycemia with chocolate, doughnuts, or other high-fat sugary foods, or with slowly absorbed carbohydrates (such as whole-grain breads or legumes), as they do not act rapidly enough for effective treatment.

Good Sources of Carbohydrate for Hypoglycemia Treatment

ANY CARBOHYDRATES you consume during and after exercise to prevent or treat hypoglycemia should be rapidly absorbable. Try consuming any of the following for the best results:

▶ Two to three glucose tablets (8 to 12 grams of carbohydrate)
▶ One to two pieces of hard or sugary candy
▶ 4 ounces of regular soda (the only good use for regular soda!)
▶ 8 ounces of juice diluted one to one with water for better absorption
▶ 8 ounces of a sports drink (most of these drinks contain 6 to 9 grams of carbohydrate per 8 ounces)
▶ 8 ounces of skim milk
▶ Two to three graham crackers or six saltines
▶ 2 tablespoons (approximately 1/4 cup) of raisins

Blood glucose monitoring. Prevention of either hypoglycemia or **hyperglycemia** during exercise is essential for feeling good and getting the most out of your activities. The key to preventing either condition is frequent monitoring and quick action to correct your BG levels. In general, for new or unusual activities, you will need to test more frequently to maintain BG control—testing before, possibly during, and after exercise—until you get a better idea of how to prevent BG fluctuations before they occur. With regular testing, you should be able to establish a pattern that allows you to figure out what your body will need for a given activity.

Carbohydrate intake. A recommendation from the **American Diabetes Association (ADA)** states that you should ingest carbohydrates if your preexercise BG level is less than 100 mg/dl (5.5 mM); however, this recommendation only applies to people with type 2 diabetes who are taking supplemental insulin injections. If you are using diet or oral diabetic medications alone, you're not likely to develop hypoglycemia, and you will not likely need any extra carbohydrates. If you're taking insulin, though, it's recommended that you ingest at least 15 grams of carbohydrate prior to exercise for a starting BG level of 100 mg/dl or lower, the exact quantity dependent on other variables such as when the injected insulin peaks and how long your activity is going to last. In all cases, you'll need fewer carbohydrates, if any, to do short, intense exercise. Alternately, if you use an **insulin pump**, you may simply choose to reduce or eliminate your basal infusion of insulin during exercise rather than eat extra carbohydrate.

Hyperglycemia. Should you exercise when your BG level is high? Technically, any BG reading in excess of 125 mg/dl (6.9 mM) qualifies as hyperglycemia, but your exercise responses will likely be normal up until your BG levels are twice as high or higher, or above 250 mg/dl (13.9 mM). Although very uncommon in type 2 diabetes, **ketosis** (a state of metabolic acidosis detected by **ketones** in the urine) may develop in people with limited or no insulin production. If it does, you should not exercise until you get rid of the ketones, as they indicate that your body is too deficient in insulin, which will likely cause your BG level to rise even more if you exercise. If you're somewhat hyperglycemic right after eating and you already took an insulin injection (maybe not a high enough dose), though, your BG levels will likely still decrease during extended exercise because enough insulin will be in your body to help bring it down during the activity, and you shouldn't have too many ketones if you haven't had high BG levels for long.

Dehydration. If you're exercising with any elevation in BG levels, take care to drink enough water, as it will be easy for you to get dehydrated. Elevated sugars can increase your water losses through excessive urination, so your risk of losing extra fluids is greater with poorly controlled BG levels. Exercising itself compounds the risk by increasing sweating (thus loss of water), which can rapidly compound a dehydrated state. Since exercising during hot weather can be especially dangerous for older individuals—who may not release heat as effectively as younger adults—adequate fluid replacement and frequent rest need to be high priorities.

Hydration Tips for Exercise

- ▶ Drink cool, plain water during and following exercise, especially during warmer weather, and take frequent breaks to have a chance to cool down, preferably out of the heat and direct sunlight.
- ▶ Drink only when you feel thirsty and don't force yourself to drink more than the amount of fluid that satisfies your thirst—or water intoxication may result.
- ▶ To know how much fluid to replace after exercise, weigh yourself before and after a prolonged activity and only replace up to the weight you have lost (1 liter of water weighs 1 kilogram, or 2.2 pounds).
- ▶ If you prefer fluids with some flavor, try flavored waters, sports drinks that have no added carbohydrates or calories (such as Champion Lyte), or Crystal Light (with a pinch of salt if you want it to taste more like a sports drink).
- ▶ Drink regular sports drinks (containing glucose) only when you need some carbohydrate to prevent or treat hypoglycemia during physical activities.

A few words of warning about hydrating. It's actually easier to harm yourself with excessive fluid intake than with **dehydration** during exercise. If you drink too much water and other fluids during exercise, you'll increase your risk of diluting the sodium content of your blood, potentially causing a medical condition known as **hyponatremia**, or water intoxication, and putting you at risk for seizures, coma, and even death. While the ADA recommends adequate hydration prior to exercise (17 ounces of fluid taken two hours before exercise) with fluids consumed early and frequently to cover sweat losses during exercise—or the maximal amount of fluid you can tolerate—updated guidelines are definitely needed. To avoid overhydrating, you should start drinking only when you actually feel thirsty. The only exception would be for people with poorly controlled diabetes, since they may have an elevated thirst threshold (meaning that they don't feel thirsty as quickly, even when dehydrated); if that applies to you, start drinking small amounts of water as soon as you start sweating.

Preventing dehydration without overloading on fluids is an individual balancing act. You should not be gaining weight during a physical activity. You will be sweating and losing water in other ways, so your weight should really go down (albeit temporarily, until you rehydrate). Replace only the weight that you have lost. Later on, after exercise, continue to use thirst as your guide, rehydrating with water or other noncaloric fluids; however, if you have consumed a lot of fluid during an activity, wait until you start to urinate before you drink any more.

As for whether you should drink water, sports drinks, or other fluids, it depends on your BG needs. For shorter activities (lasting an hour or less), plain water is fine—unless you need some extra carbohydrate to prevent your BG level from dropping too much, in which case you can drink a sports drink such as Gatorade or Powerade. You don't need to worry about replacing electrolytes, such as sodium, potassium, and chloride, unless you are exercising outdoors in hot weather for more than two hours at a time; even then, you can usually wait to replace electrolytes naturally with food the next time you eat.

THE BOTTOM LINE ON STEP 1
Get Down to Basics

▶ You can't blame diabetes on your genes alone; your lifestyle choices matter more.

▶ Exercise truly is the best "medicine" for your diabetes—and whatever else ails you.

▶ Being active can prevent most diabetic complications, including an early death.

▶ Your excess body fat is not the direct or only possible cause of all your BG problems.

▶ Small reductions in body weight (10 to 15 pounds for most people) will bring you almost all the health benefits of being at a normal weight.

▶ If you have lost weight, you're likely to keep it off only with regular exercise.

▶ Your insulin sensitivity will greatly improve with any regular physical activity, no matter whether you lose any weight or not.

▶ It is possible to be physically fit even if you're overweight.

▶ Only exercise is truly effective at helping you lose "bad" visceral fat from your abdomen.

▶ You can exercise safely and effectively with diabetes if you follow a few simple rules.

As you can see from this first step, you need to know as much as possible about your diabetes and your body in order to get the most out of your physical activities. Without the additional caloric expenditure and other physical benefits that exercise provides, dieters are doomed to regain their lost weight (and more), and the rest of us can look forward to fat-weight gain in the future.

In the second step to diabetes fitness, I will discuss what types of exercise are especially important for you to do, and why.

DIABETES FITNESS PLAN STEP 1
in a Nutshell

YOUR LIFESTYLE choices matter most in controlling your diabetes or pre-diabetes. The goal is to improve your insulin sensitivity and glucose use, and physical activity and increased fitness are best suited to help you accomplish this goal, no matter how much you weigh.

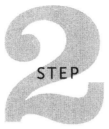

STEP 2

Get Up and Get Moving

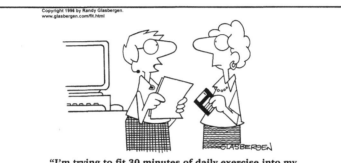

"I'm trying to fit 30 minutes of daily exercise into my busy schedule. Today I took 120 fifteen-second walks."

H AS YOUR DOCTOR told you to be more physically active, but failed to provide any specifics other than to "exercise more"? If so, you're not alone. According to recent research, 52 percent of doctors tell their diabetic patients to exercise, but only 14 percent actually "prescribe" it by giving them a specific exercise plan to follow. The medical profession's stance really should be that exercise is an integral part of your daily regimen, just like brushing your teeth. I firmly believe that not only is it not optional, but it should be prescribed to everyone, along with dietary improvements and, as appropriate, diabetic medications.

Although exercising involves much more work than making adjustments to your diet or just taking medications to control your diabetes, it is well worth the effort for myriad health-related reasons. This section will teach you what you need to know about including appropriate physical activity in your daily regimen to achieve optimal health and fitness. In addition, it discusses how to exercise safely and effectively if you have any diabetic complications, other health concerns, or physical limitations.

Do you need to see your doctor first?

If you haven't been very active lately, do you need to see your doctor before you begin exercising more? Well, it depends. Medical clearance for low-level exercise is usually not necessary. However, for more vigorous exercise, seeing your doctor before you begin is a good idea. The more risk factors that you have for heart disease, the greater your chance of having a cardiovascular problem during exercise, and prior knowledge of what you need to watch out for could be crucial. That is not to say that you should avoid exercising if you do have some pre-existing cardiovascular problems; on the contrary, regular moderate to vigorous activity can actually reduce your risk of a heart attack, even if you have already had one.

You May Want to See Your Doctor First If You . . .

- ▶ Are planning on participating in moderate to strenuous activities, not just mild ones
- ▶ Are over 35 years of age
- ▶ Have been diagnosed with type 1 diabetes for more than 15 years or type 2 for more than 10 years
- ▶ Know you have heart disease, a strong family history of heart disease, or high cholesterol or lipid levels
- ▶ Have poor circulation in your feet or legs (or lower-leg pain while walking)
- ▶ Have retinopathy (diabetic eye disease), **nephropathy** (kidney disease), or neuropathy (numbness, burning, tingling, or loss of sensation in your feet and/or dizziness when going from sitting to standing)
- ▶ Have not consistently been in good control of your BG levels

Most people with type 2 diabetes should undergo a thorough medical exam prior to starting most exercise programs; such an exam should include a physical exam, urinalysis, kidney function testing, serum lipid evaluation, electrolyte balance, and exercise stress testing. The point of such testing is primarily to screen for the presence of any diabetes-related complications, including heart, nerve, eye, and kidney disease. While having such health problems does not automatically preclude you from exercising, doing so safely and effectively with any of these complications may require special accommodations or precautions that will be discussed in detail later in this step.

Get moving with extra steps

"Physical activity" means so much more than just planned activities. By this I mean that even standing, talking, and fidgeting use up extra calories and can make a difference in your body weight. In tracking lean and obese people for 10 days, researchers observed that the overweight, self-proclaimed "couch potatoes" stayed seated for about 2.5 hours longer per day than their leaner counterparts, amounting to a lower calorie expenditure of about 350 calories per day—the caloric equivalent of about 36 pounds a year. Thus, just staying on your feet more can have a beneficial impact on your body weight.

Beliefs about exercise have changed dramatically over the past decade, especially as so many people have begun to gain extra body fat. Scientists and health-care providers used to believe that exercise had to be vigorous to bestow meaningful health benefits, but more recently, a study conducted at Harvard found that, for adult women at least, moderate walking decreased their risk for developing diabetes as effectively as more vigorous activities. Simply being physically active during your leisure time—particularly if you're doing longer or more intense activities—also reduces your diabetes risk.

President's Challenge: Helpful Ideas to Get Active

▶ Use a push mower to mow the lawn.
▶ Go for a walk in a nearby park.
▶ Take the stairs instead of an elevator.
▶ Bike to work, to run errands, or to visit friends.
▶ Clean out the garage or the attic.
▶ Walk with a friend over the lunch hour.
▶ Volunteer to become a coach or referee.
▶ Sign up for a group exercise class.
▶ Join a softball league.
▶ Park at the farthest end of the lot.

The President's Challenge;
www.presidentschallenge.org/tools_to_help/ten_ideas.aspx

Taking extra steps throughout the day will be well worth the effort. Additional walking can be added into your daily routine more easily than you might imagine. For example, try taking a flight of steps instead of the elevator or an escalator whenever possible, or at least walk up or down the escalator instead of standing while it does the work for you. If going up steps is too hard, then start with just walking down. Another good idea is to hide the remote to your TV so that you have to get up to change the channel manually. You might even think about washing the dishes yourself instead of letting the dishwasher do the work. Another good idea is to walk around for five minutes after every half hour of being sedentary.

TIP
10

NO MATTER YOUR WEIGHT

AS FAR as your health is concerned, what really matters is expending those extra calories any way that you can. To start moving more, consider walking: simply increase the number of steps that you take during the day and/or add in planned walks.

As recently as June 2005, a study in Diabetes Care confirmed that, if you have type 2 diabetes and you increase your aerobic activity by thirty-eight minutes per day—walking just an extra 4,400 steps, or about 2.2 miles—you'll experience noteworthy reductions in your BG, total cholesterol, **triglycerides** (blood fats), and blood pressure even if you don't lose weight. Not surprisingly, if you add even more leisure-time physical activity—such as more than 10,000 steps a day—you can enjoy even greater improvements in your health. More activity can even decrease your risk of having a **stroke** by at least 25 percent, even if you have diabetes. As an added bonus, the participants in that study also reduced their risk of heart disease more than twofold and their annual medical costs by an average of $288.

Count your daily steps for motivation

Walking is the most popular leisure-time physical activity among adults, followed by gardening and yard work. Generally, walking expends about 1 calorie per kilogram (kg) of body weight (pounds divided by 2.2 equals a kilogram) per kilometer (about 0.6 miles) when you walk at a speed of 2 to 4 miles per hour; for a person weighing 60 kg (130 lb), about 100 calories are used up per mile. Depending on the length of your stride, about 2,000 steps equals a mile; if you're overweight, you will expend well more than 100 extra calories because of your larger body size. Incredibly, just taking those 2,000 extra steps a day can make the difference between gaining and losing weight (or at least not gaining any more).

If motivation is your biggest problem, make a game out of trying to count how many steps you take or set daily goals for yourself. Instructing sedentary, overweight women to walk 10,000 steps per day (monitored by a pedometer) has proven to be more effective at increasing their daily exercise than asking them to walk 30 minutes most days of the week. Based on the 10,000 step study mentioned previously, it appears that we could all benefit immensely from taking at least 10,000 steps each day. If nothing else, becoming more conscious of how active you are (or are not) during the day may spur you to add in more steps whenever possible. You may want to consider investing in an inexpensive pedometer for additional motivation. Keep in mind that, on average, 3,100 to 4,000 pedometer-determined steps are equivalent to 30 minutes of moderate-intensity walking.

Finding Motivation in Counting Your Daily Steps

THE ADA sponsors Club Ped, an online group (www.diabetes.org/ClubPed/index.jsp) that you can join to keep track of your steps, your progress, and your step goals. All you need to get started is a pedometer. In addition, a national campaign called "America on the Move" (www.americaonthemove.org) advocates a minimum increase of 2,000 steps per day for everyone and offers a free online step tracker.

Many other pedometer-based walking programs can be accessed online at Web sites, including AccuSplit pedometer company, www.accustep10000.org, and StepTracker.com, www.steptracker.com. You can also purchase inexpensive pedometers through sporting-goods stores or order them online from various Web sites, including www.americaonthemove.org, www.accusplit.com, www.digiwalker.com, www.walk4life.com, www.steps-to-health.org, and www.pedometersusa.com.

A few tips on pedometer use: if you clip a pedometer somewhere on the front of your waistband and it does not appear to be accurate, try placing it at the small of your back (some pedometers are less effective if you have extra fat around your waist). Some models can actually be placed in your pocket (e.g., Omron

Healthcare pedometers) or attached around your knee. Pedometers vary greatly in terms of accuracy and performance. While you may like ones with bells and whistles like calorie counters and distance trackers, all you really need is a pedometer that will accurately count the number of steps you take. Calorie counts are notoriously inaccurate (even on conditioning machines), and distance trackers depend on having an accurate measurement of the length of your stride (which then can't be varied) to make their calculations. Go for simplicity but accuracy in step counters. Recommended models are Accusplit (the simplest model being the X120, with more features on the Eagle and Alliance models), Walk4Life (Neo Walkin' Buddy or W4L Classic models), Yamax (SW200), and Omron (HJ-112 Premium) pedometers.

Other unstructured activities count, too

Getting yourself motivated to be more physically active is not nearly as hard as you might think. The main thing is that you start to think more broadly about what constitutes exercise. Stop trying to find the closest parking spot, using remote controls for everything in your house, and waiting for the elevator when you could be using the stairs. Just adding a dozen steps here and there while doing household chores, yard work, or errands, along with standing, making extra arm movements, stretching, and other general body movement can easily add up to a substantial amount of energy expended over the course of the day and suffice to prevent insulin resistance and weight gain.

Maybe walking is not your cup of tea, and you'd rather take a bike ride around the nearest park. That's okay, too, but keep in mind that cycling expends only about a third of the energy you use walking the same distance, so you would have to bike about three miles to equal walking just one. Doing either activity, though, you're still expending calories, which is the important thing.

In reality, any exercise you do during the day counts. Now that you know that participation in intense activities (done at more than 60 percent of maximal aerobic capacity, such as jogging) is not necessary for optimal health and fitness, the world of physical activity is wide open. Pick your favorite leisure-time activity—golfing, gardening, mowing the lawn, or walking the dog—and do it a total of 30 to 45 minutes per day (for as little as ten minutes at a time). Even if your fitness level is not increased much, your overall health will benefit. Your new goal is simply to be as physically active as possible during the day to maximize caloric expenditure and BG use.

It's time for you to start taking the stairs instead of the elevator (and doing so several times a day). Some additional ways to add in more unstructured activities are listed in the following table, but be sure to think up more of your own—you know best your unique situation and interests.

Easy Ways to Add Unstructured Exercise

- Add as many additional steps as possible (a minimum of 2,000) every day by walking whenever and wherever you can.
- Whenever you have ten free minutes, walk around instead of sitting down—or at least stand up.
- Always take the stairs instead of the elevator or escalator.
- Do physical chores around the house, such as cleaning, sweeping, mopping, vacuuming, and washing dishes (even if you have a dishwasher).
- Rake leaves in the yard or shovel snow.
- Go shopping for groceries or window-shopping at the nearest mall.
- Put on some music and dance around your house.
- Set up a basketball hoop in your driveway, or walk to the nearest neighborhood school and use theirs.
- Take the dog out for a daily walk (it needs exercise, too!).
- Get up and move around for a few minutes after every 30 minutes of a sedentary activity.
- Walk around while talking on the telephone instead of sitting down.
- Hide the remotes for the TV, stereo, and other devices.
- Walk in place, dance, move around, or even just stand up while watching TV—at least during the commercial breaks.
- Invest in a rebounder (mini-trampoline) and jump on it while watching TV.
- Limit your TV and computer use to no more than two hours per day, or at least reduce your use by a minimum of 30 minutes daily.

Choosing planned activities: cardio, strength, toning, and flexibility

Now that you're moving your body more, you might want to consider adding in some other types of activities to maximize your fitness and diabetes control. Before you do so, though, it's important to consider how various structured activities can benefit your health and BG levels. For instance, stretching and other flexibility activities are important in limiting flexibility losses as you age, but aren't as effective in using up a lot of BG. On the other hand, prolonged cardiovascular (aerobic) workouts generally lower BG levels. To help you decide what is best for you, the benefits and potential drawbacks of various types of activities are discussed in more detail in the following section; specific exercises and sample exercise plans are described in more detail in the next fitness step.

Cardio workouts get your heart going

Aerobic, or "cardio," exercise gets your heart working harder. As your blood is pumped faster, it must be oxygenated in less time as it passes by your lungs, which in turn quickens your breathing. Consequently, aerobic exercise strengthens your heart and boosts the levels of your healthy cholesterol. Lower-impact aerobic exercises include mild walking, swimming, cycling, tai chi, and the like. Higher-impact aerobic exercise includes running, tennis, and aerobic dance classes.

Moderate walking is likely the best medicine for both the prevention and treatment of type 2 diabetes and for your overall health, and it has the added bonus of being more sustainable over a lifetime than many other activities. The surgeon general recently recommended moderate amounts of daily, aerobic physical activity for people of all ages including 30 minutes of moderate activities (like brisk walking) or shorter sessions—15 to 20 minutes—of more intense exercise, including jogging or playing basketball. Of course, engaging in even more total physical activity may offer you additional benefits—but only up to a point. The incidence of **overuse injuries**, such as inflamed tendons (tendonitis) and stress fractures in bones, soars when you do more than 60 to 90 minutes of hard exercise daily.

TIP

11

NO MATTER YOUR WEIGHT

IF YOU'RE overweight, you may have special concerns about doing structured exercise routines. You may become so self-conscious about your body during such activities that it prevents you from wanting to participate at all, or the activities may seem too difficult. If this sounds like you, it's especially important for you to find activities that you perceive as enjoyable to have any hope of continuing with them. Try out a few different activities until you find one or two that you really like. It will be well worth your extra effort.

Ideally, structured aerobic exercise programs should involve activities that allow you to move your whole body over the greatest distance possible to maximize your energy use. However, although walking and jogging fall into this category of activity, most overweight adults will find jogging and running either too difficult or simply unenjoyable. Try tricking yourself into walking by incorporating it into other activities—such as walking farther than you need to when you go shopping. Walking can be the gateway to more vigorous exercise, which can further increase your overall health benefits. Your self-confidence may improve once you start a walking program, which may lead you to start including additional physical activities into your life. You might even want to try out ballroom dancing, cycling, low-impact aerobics classes, or other forms of aerobic exercise. Remember to take advantage of any strong physical attributes that you have—such as stronger legs from carrying around your extra body weight.

TIP
12

NO MATTER YOUR WEIGHT

EXTRA FAT stored under the skin acts to insulate you and keep you warmer in the pool, which is an advantage in pools heated to 80° F or less, since heat losses through the skin in water are usually much greater than in air. If you are overweight, then, swimming or aquatic classes may be a good choice for you. Also, the water serves to hide your figure, which can decrease any inhibition you may feel being more plainly visible during other activities.

Strength and toning moves keep you from losing it

Strength training is imperative to maintain the amount of muscle you currently have, to gain more, and to prevent losses of muscle and strength as you age. Inactivity also accelerates your loss of muscle mass (the old "Use it or lose it" adage is also true in this case). Even though aerobic training can help, only the **muscle fibers** that you recruit and use regularly will be maintained over time; unfortunately, moderate walking does not bring all of your muscle fibers into play. Only harder workouts can do that.

Muscle fibers run the spectrum from being very aerobic (slow-twitch fibers) to being mainly recruited for heavy lifting or near-maximal exercise (fast-twitch fibers); all types of fibers can exist within a single muscle. How many and which muscles you recruit during an activity depends on how much force your muscles have to produce. For example, for easy work, you use only the very aerobic (slow) fibers in the muscles you're using. However, if you increase your workload, you'll be recruiting not just the slow ones, but also some of the intermediate-speed fibers. To do a maximal weight lift or all-out sprint, you'll be recruiting all of the ones we've discussed so far, plus your very fastest fibers, which are capable of producing the most power in the shortest amount of time.

It's easy to tell when those fastest fibers are being recruited, because their work is fueled primarily by our first two energy systems, the phosphagens and the lactic acid system. If a heavy lift takes you only one to two seconds to complete, then you invariably just use the ATP (part of the phosphagen system) that you already had stored in your muscle ready for use. For activities lasting longer than 10 seconds but less than a minute (such as a resistance-training exercise), you should recognize the uncomfortable, "burning" sensation in your working muscles as the lactic acid system (which breaks down muscle glycogen) coming into play. This sensation is not harmful to your muscles, and it's an excellent means of knowing whether you're recruiting all of the faster muscle fibers that you want to keep.

The addition of resistance training can bestow extra health benefits. Such training increases muscle mass, which can enhance both your insulin action and your round-the-clock resting energy expenditure (and, thus, glycemic control), not to mention **self-esteem** and feelings of accomplishment. You will also experience measurable increases in strength in as short a time as one to two weeks (from neural changes, which occur before increases in muscle size), which will serve as additional motivation. Furthermore, major strength gains are possible even if you train as infrequently as one day a week.

Strength gains are the key to preventing injuries, particularly from falling, which occurs more often as people age. Increases in strength can also prevent the frailty that so often accompanies old age, enhance your ability to care for yourself, and improve your physical and mental health. Some people may be confined to a wheelchair simply because getting up out of it is too difficult, but the increased strength gained from resistance work can enable them to return to doing more activities out of their wheelchairs.

Living with chronic pain is also a reality for many people, and strength gains have been shown to alleviate pain associated with muscle weakness—such as is often the case with lower back pain. Humans do not have the structural advantage of walking on all fours; when you walk, your lower back must bear the brunt of your body's weight. Our lower backs have also come to bear much of the increasing stress of daily living in a modern world, including poor posture, lack of exercise, and weight gain. As we become more sedentary, stress on our lower backs is only increased, since sitting is, in fact, an unnatural position. In addition to assuming a better posture, exercising more, and losing some of your belly fat, specifically working to strengthen your lower back is the best way to prevent lower back pain and injuries.

Flexibility work makes your joints mobile

Working on your flexibility also helps prevent injuries and is doubly important for anyone with diabetes. We're all becoming less flexible over time—just compare the limberness of an infant with the inflexibility of an older adult—so some loss of flexibility is to be expected. However, an elevated BG level by itself can speed up this loss of flexibility by binding to joint structures (collagen and the like) and causing them to become more brittle and less flexible. A loss of flexibility leads to a reduced range of motion for your joints, an increased likelihood of orthopedic injuries, and a greater risk of developing some of the joint-related problems often associated with diabetes. These include diabetic "frozen shoulder," tendonitis, trigger finger, carpal tunnel syndrome, and others.

The **American College of Sports Medicine** (ACSM) recommends that you work on your flexibility a minimum of two to three days per week, but I recommend stretching before and/or after any exercise session or any other time that your muscles start to tighten up. Depending on the exercise that I'm doing, I may stretch before (running), during (after about five minutes of swimming, when my shoulders tighten up), or after (resistance training). It doesn't seem to matter when you stretch, as long as you do it, but it's usually easier to do once you've warmed up a little. Some basic stretches to include in your routine are illustrated in the next step.

TIP
13

─────────────── **NO MATTER YOUR WEIGHT** ───────────────

TO GET the maximum benefits from stretching to minimize the loss of flexibility caused by aging and accelerated by diabetes, include stretching exercises into your new, healthier lifestyle a minimum of two or three days per week. This will also help you maximize your strength gains from any concurrent resistance exercises you may be doing.

Exercising with diabetic or other health limitations

Is your health your main excuse for not being more physically active? Whether your biggest health complaint is high blood pressure, loss of feeling in your feet, or arthritic knees, it's time to change your way of thinking. There is mounting evidence that older individuals with chronic health problems respond just as well to exercise training as their younger counterparts, yet many older people still choose not to be physically active. While it's true that 85 percent of people over the age of sixty-five have a health problem that they may view as a deterrent to exercise, diabetes should definitely not be among them, and neither should almost all of the others.

Although most everyone can exercise safely and effectively, diabetes does bring additional risks, as discussed in the preceding step. However, you can still exercise to your potential—as long as you respect your limitations. To stay safe and get the most out of your activities, follow the exercise guidelines published by the ADA. The remainder of this section will address how you can overcome other common health concerns, allowing you to be as physically active as possible.

Cardiovascular disease. If you have diabetes or prediabetes, you may also have cardiovascular disease. Remember that about a third of all people with diabetes are not even aware of having it; sadly, many of them first learn of their condition while in the hospital after suffering their first heart attack, stroke, or other cardiovascular event. Does having heart disease mean that exercise is not for you? Absolutely not. Resistance training is now recommended for everyone, even people with known cardiovascular disease who have had a heart attack or stroke.

Diabetic people in supervised cardiac-rehabilitation exercise programs engage in various forms of exercise, and you may choose to join such a program if you know you have cardiovascular disease; you may also prefer to exercise on your own. It's important to know that you're more likely to experience **angina** (chest pain) due to reduced blood flow to your heart muscle (**ischemia**) during an aerobic activity like treadmill walking than during weight training. Studies have shown that lifting a heavy weight ten to twelve times may increase your blood pressure more than aerobic work, but it doesn't raise your heart rate as much. Ironically, the higher blood pressures reached during resistance training ensure that your heart muscle gets more blood than it would during aerobic activities. If you know that you have some coronary artery blockage from plaque buildup, moderate weight training may actually be a safer activity for you than most high-intensity aerobic ones.

If you prefer aerobic activities or if you do both types, use pain as your guide. In general, if reaching a certain heart rate (in number of beats per minute, or bpm) causes you to develop chest pain during exercise, always exercise at an intensity that keeps your rate at least 10 bpm below that pain threshold. For example, if slow jogging causes you to feel angina at a heart rate of 140 bpm, then lower your exercise intensity by walking briskly instead, to keep your heart rate at 130 bpm or below at all times. In addition, be aware that a heart attack may have symptoms other than pain localized in your chest, such as pain that radiates down one arm or shoulder or your neck or that feels like bad heartburn. If you experience any unusual pain or other symptoms during or following exercise, get checked out by your doctor as soon as possible. Diabetes can also potentially cause you to experience **silent ischemia**, a reduction in blood flow to the heart muscle through the coronary blood vessels that is painless and symptom-free. If you experience a sudden, unexplained change in your ability to exercise, without any other symptoms, immediately stop exercising and consult with your physician as soon as you can to rule out silent ischemia.

Finally, diabetes can cause a cardiovascular condition known as **peripheral vascular disease (PVD)**, which reduces blood flow to your lower extremities. Some people with PVD have pain in their legs while walking or standing. If you experience these symptoms during or after physical activities and you have not yet been diagnosed with PVD, it would be best to confer with your physician to get a definite diagnosis before proceeding with your exercise program. If you do have blood-flow limitations to your lower legs and feet, you may have to choose activities that do not result in pain, such as seated exercises, water workouts, or stationary cycling.

Hypertension. In addition to improving diabetes-related health, regular aerobic exercise lessens the potential impact of most of the other cardiovascular risk factors, including elevated blood lipids (cholesterol and other blood fats), insulin resistance, obesity, and hypertension. Hypertension is associated with hyperinsulinemia, and regular physical activity can result in lower blood pressure and reduced circulating levels of insulin, making it very beneficial as far as your health is concerned.

If you have elevated blood pressure, though, it is best to avoid certain higher-intensity or heavy resistance exercises, which may cause your blood pressure to rise dangerously high and precipitate a stroke or other cardiovascular event. Activities best avoided include heavy weight training, near-maximal exercise of any type, activities that require intense, sustained contractions of the upper body, such as water-skiing or windsurfing, or any exercise for which you must hold your breath.

Peripheral neuropathy and lower limb ulcers. Loss of sensation in your feet or hands is called **peripheral neuropathy**, and if you have it, your risk of damaging your feet, in particular during exercise, increases greatly. Peripheral nerve damage can blunt the usual symptoms of pain or discomfort resulting from impact on your feet or friction and pressure from footwear, making it easy to develop a blister or sore on your foot without being aware of it. In some cases, a simple blister can progress to a full-blown infected abscess or ulcer and ultimately result in a lower-limb amputation if not properly cared for in time.

If you have lost feeling in your feet, the ADA recommends that you use shoes with silica gel or air midsoles (the middle section of the shoe that provides the most stability and shock absorption), as well as polyester or cotton-polyester socks to prevent the formation of blisters and to keep your feet dry during physical activities. (Pure cotton socks tend to get wet and stay wet, which may promote damage to your feet.) It is also imperative that you (or someone else, if you are not able to) check your feet daily for signs of trauma and treat them aggressively to prevent any worsening of the problem.

If you have lost feeling in your feet or already have an ulcer that has not yet healed, it may also be a good idea to switch to activities such as swimming or stationary cycling that minimize the trauma to your lower extremities. Walking, jogging, and other such activities require you to place your full body weight on your feet. Good **non-weight-bearing exercises** include anything aquatic (swimming, pool walking, water aerobics, and the like), upper-body exercises (rowing, arm crank ergometers, and other upper-body work), chair exercises, stationary cycling, yoga, and abdominal work, among others. These activities, in addition to minimizing potential foot problems while allowing you to remain active, also improve your body tone, balance, and awareness of your lower extremities.

Exercise doesn't appear to have the capacity to reverse peripheral neuropathy, but it can slow its progression and prevent further loss of fitness from occurring due to inactivity, and it may also improve circulation in your lower legs and feet enough to help prevent ulcers from forming. However, your neuropathy may have progressed to the point that you have some physical difficulties and limitations in exercising; for example, your peripheral nerve damage may cause dull, shooting, or throbbing pain in your extremities after you go for a walk or engage in other weight-bearing activities. If you ever experience this type of painful neuropathy due to a certain activity, then it's best to limit that activity in the future and switch to others that don't cause you lasting pain or discomfort.

Autonomic neuropathy. Other diabetes-related complications may also require some modifications in your exercise program. For example, if you have damage to your central nervous system (**autonomic neuropathy**), you're more likely to experience silent ischemia. This could result in a "silent" or undetected heart attack. Your chances of dying suddenly during exercise from such an event are high once your heart has become unresponsive to nerve impulses due to autonomic neuropathy—especially if you have underlying heart disease.

If severe, this complication may also make it harder for you to change your body position (e.g., going from sitting to standing or from lying to sitting) without experiencing orthostatic hypotension, which can result in lightheadedness or fainting. You're also more likely to overheat and get dehydrated. If this type of nerve damage affects your ability to digest and absorb foods (known as "gastroparesis"), any carbohydrate you eat to treat a low BG reaction during exercise might be more slowly absorbed, and your hypoglycemia might become more severe as a result. Finally, this complication may cause you to have an elevated heart rate at rest (for example, 100 bpm instead of the normal 72 beats), and it can keep your heart from beating as fast as it should once you start to exercise.

If you have been diagnosed with autonomic nerve damage, take a conservative approach to exercise. Try to avoid rapid changes in movement that may result in fainting and take a longer time (10 minutes or more) to warm up and cool down, particularly when you're doing strenuous activities. Drink extra fluids during exercise, and avoid being continuously active for long periods during hotter weather conditions. Also, avoid eating a large meal before exercise as it could result in delayed emptying of food from your stomach. Eat only small portions beforehand, and treat hypoglycemia with easily absorbed glucose tablets before BG levels become too low (when they reach 100 mg/dl) to prevent severe hyperglycemia. Finally, monitor your exercise by some means other than your heart rate alone, since it may no longer rise as much as expected or be the best way to monitor your exercise intensity.

Diabetic eye disease. People with diabetes are prone to developing all sorts of eye complications, including cataracts and retinopathy. While cataracts can obscure your vision and make participation in certain activities (such as cycling outdoors) more dangerous, they're not usually considered a barrier to participation in physical pursuits. On the other hand, more severe forms of eye disease, such as proliferative diabetic retinopathy, cause your eyes to form weak, abnormal blood vessels in the back of the eye (the retina) that can break, tear, or bleed into the vitreous fluid in the center of your eye, filling it with blood that can obscure vision temporarily or permanently. If you have severe eye disease, you will need to make greater changes to your exercise regimen to prevent bleeding into your eye.

While exercise itself has not been shown to accelerate the proliferative process, certain precautions may be needed to prevent intra-ocular hemorrhages or retinal tears. If your eye disease is only mild or moderate, with no active bleeds, then you should simply avoid activities that dramatically increase the blood pressure inside your eyes, such as heavy weight lifting or activities during which your head is lower than your heart. If you have moderate to severe diabetic eye disease, you'll want to avoid all jumping, jarring, or breath-holding activities, as they increase the pressure inside your eyes and can cause more bleeding and increase your risk of retinal tears or retinal detachment. Activities best avoided include boxing, competitive contact sports (such as basketball and football), jogging, high-impact aerobics, most racket sports, and heavy weight lifting. If you have an active retinal hemorrhage or notice sudden, dramatic changes in your sight, stop any activity you are doing immediately and check with your eye doctor for further guidance.

Precautions for Exercising with Diabetes and/or Its Complications

- ▶ Have a BG meter accessible to check your BG level before, possibly during, and/or after exercise, or if you have any symptoms of low sugars.
- ▶ Immediately treat any low BG during or following exercise with easily absorbed carbohydrates like glucose tablets or regular soft drinks, which you should keep handy.
- ▶ Inform your exercise partner(s) about your diabetes, and show them how to administer glucose or another carbohydrate to you should you need assistance in treating a low.
- ▶ Stay properly hydrated with frequent intake of small amounts of cool water.
- ▶ Consult with your physician prior to exercising with any of the following conditions:
  - Proliferative retinopathy or current retinal hemorrhage
  - Neuropathy (nerve damage), either peripheral or autonomic
  - Foot injuries (including ulcers)
  - High blood pressure
  - Serious illness or infection
- ▶ Seek immediate medical attention for chest pain or any pain that radiates down your arm, jaw, or neck.
- ▶ If you have hypertension, avoid activities that cause large increases in your blood pressure, such as heavy resistance work, head-down exercises, and anything that forces you to hold your breath.
- ▶ Wear proper footwear, and check your feet daily for signs of trauma such as blisters, redness, or other irritation.
- ▶ Immediately stop exercising if you experience bleeding into your eyes caused by active proliferative retinopathy.
- ▶ Wear a diabetes medic alert bracelet or necklace with your physician's name and contact information on it.

Diabetic kidney disease. Luckily, exercise does not appear to worsen nephropathy—otherwise known as kidney disease—which is common to diabetes. Intense or prolonged exercise would not usually be recommended for you if you have overt kidney disease, but only because your exercise capacity is likely to be limited. Light to moderate exercise is fine, though, and even patients requiring dialysis can exercise—even during their dialysis treatments, if they want to—with no ill effects. If you are undergoing dialysis, exercise would only be advised against if the levels of certain substances in your blood (hematocrit, calcium, or potassium) become unbalanced as a result of the treatments. People who have undergone kidney transplants due to end-stage kidney disease can safely exercise six to eight weeks after surgery, once they are stable and free of signs of rejection of the new kidney.

You may not be aware that exercise itself can increase the excretion in your urine of protein and/or microalbumin which are traditionally used by your doctor as indicators of kidney problems. For your peace of mind, and to prevent false conclusions, abstain from exercising on any day that you are collecting your urine for either of these tests so that your results will not be erroneously skewed and misinterpreted as evidence of kidney damage or disease progression.

Exercising with excess body weight. Carrying around extra body fat can pose a formidable challenge to being physically active. Excess weight alone can often keep you from wanting or being able to participate in sports or other physical pursuits, thus potentially creating a catch-22 for weight management and self-care. For example, choosing not to participate in physical activities due to your excessive body size lowers your daily calorie expenditure, which causes you to potentially gain more weight. At the same time, being sedentary makes you lose muscle mass, making you weaker and robbing you of any incentive to become more active.

TIP
14
NO MATTER YOUR WEIGHT

IF YOU'RE currently sedentary and overweight, you may be resistant to trying exercise. Ease into being more active by taking small steps in that direction. First try doing activities that don't require you to carry around your full body weight, such as swimming, other aquatic activities or classes in a swimming pool, seated exercises, stretching, and light resistance training. As your fitness level gradually increases, you may find yourself able to try new activities that you were previously incapable of doing.

Start out slowly, so that you neither injure yourself nor cause yourself to lose motivation. Walking more is a great way to start, but it is not for everyone, so don't hesitate to try out different low-intensity activities until you find the ones that are most enjoyable for you.

You can choose to get moving simply by doing non-weight-bearing exercises, such as any swimming pool–based activity, stationary cycling, and other activities done off your feet. Many exercises can be done seated, and there are countless articles, books, videos, and DVDs on the subject. Many of the stretches and resistance activities given in the next fitness step can also be modified slightly to work from a sitting or lying position, if that makes them easier for you to do.

Exercise Videos and DVDs for Everyone

A WIDE selection of videotapes and DVDs demonstrating various physical activities, including exercise routines to be done in a chair or wheelchair, are available from a variety of sources. You can find materials for aerobic workouts, strength training, flexibility moves, yoga, and more. In addition to finding them at local sporting-goods stores and national chains, some online sources to peruse for workout videos are the following: Stronger Seniors (www.strongerseniors.com), Active Videos (www.activevideos.com), Just About Fitness (www.justabout fitness.com), and Collage Video (www.collagevideo.com). In addition, three workouts highly recommended by About.com include: (1) Jodi Stolove, *Chair Dancing through the Decades* (2004) and *Chair Dancing around the World* (2004); (2) *Tai-Chi Exercises for Seniors* (1998); and (3) *Doctor's Senior Exercise* (1998). Try out various ones to see which works best for you.

Orthopedic problems and arthritis. Simply by having diabetes, you already have a high risk of both joint-related injuries and overuse problems like tendonitis. You may therefore find that adopting a more moderate exercise like walking rather than a more vigorous one like running makes more sense, since you'll have less potential for joint trauma with the former. Diabetic frozen shoulder, "trigger finger," and other acute joint problems can also come on with no warning and for no readily apparent reason. The best defense is to prevent all of these injuries with good BG control, in addition to doing flexibility exercises that help emphasize and maintain a full range of motion around all your joints.

Arthritis is also more common in people with type 2 diabetes due to the extra body weight most of them are carrying around. Lower extremity joints (the hip, knee, and ankle) are most often affected, and, when present, osteoarthritis can severely limit your ability to exercise. However, research has clearly shown that exercise is an effective means of managing arthritis, even the more severe rheumatoid type. Get started with some basic range-of-motion exercises to increase your joint mobility, and then move on to specific resistance work. You will derive immense benefit from both improving joint flexibility and increasing the strength of your muscles surrounding any affected joints.

Not surprisingly, the number one reason why older adults, many of whom have arthritis, require assisted living is not the arthritis, but insufficient leg strength, which leaves them unable to get up out of a chair, climb stairs, or function on their own. If these people start exercising—particularly doing resistance and flexibility training—they are much more likely to be able to care for themselves, carry their own groceries, play with their grandchildren, and, most importantly, live independently.

If you have arthritic knees or hips, walking may be too uncomfortable or painful. Your best option is to try non-weight-bearing activities, such as "walking" in a pool (with or without a flotation belt around your waist), aqua aerobics, lap swimming, recumbent stationary cycling, upper-body exercises, seated aerobic workouts, and resistance activities.

TIP
15

NO MATTER YOUR WEIGHT

CARRYING AROUND extra body weight is harder on the joints in your lower extremities (i.e., your hips, knees, and ankles). Try out different activities until you find the ones that are the most comfortable for you to do, and stick with those. In addition, make certain to include adequate warmup and cool-down periods, along with flexibility and strength exercises.

No matter what physical activity you choose to do, start out slowly and progress gradually—using pain as your guide. If you have extremely arthritic joints or flare-ups of pain, concentrate on non-weight-bearing activities. After exercising, you may want to apply ice to your arthritic joints (particularly your knees) for 15 to 20 minutes to reduce swelling and help prevent soreness, and you may additionally benefit from taking nonsteroidal anti-inflammatory medications such as aspirin or ibuprofen to temporarily lessen any discomfort related to the exercise.

Another strategy that can help prevent and treat all orthopedic problems (both increased arthritic pain and more general injuries) is the concept of **cross training**, in which stressing different muscles and using varying joints from day to day can prevent problems with overuse and keep all of your joints moving more freely. I'll discuss cross training in more detail in the following fitness step.

Other physical disabilities. Having a disability that leaves you with limited mobility or in a wheelchair is not an acceptable excuse for being completely inactive. In fact, research has shown that working just your upper body can increase your mobility as you gain enhanced upper-body strength, endurance, and flexibility. Any type of activity can also give you most of exercise's health benefits, regardless of the wheelchair.

Many organizations are dedicated to assisting people with physical disabilities, helping them to live healthier lives that include physical activity. One such organization is the National Center on Physical Activity and Disability (NCPAD). The NCPAD encourages persons with disabilities to participate in regular physical activity as a means of promoting healthy lifestyles and preventing development of secondary health problems. Their slogan is, "Exercise is for everybody and every person can gain some health benefit from being more physically active." They can give you information about leisure activities, health and exercise programs, other resources listed by state (such as local fitness programs in your area), equipment adaptations, and applied products listed by company. On their Web site (www.ncpad.org), you can also find out about wheelchair sports, including boccie, bowling, golf, hunting, skiing, tai chi, and tennis. If you're more the adventurous type, check out the National Sports Center for the Disabled (www.nscd.org), which is one of the largest outdoor therapeutic recreation agencies in the world. Each year with their assistance, thousands of children and adults with disabilities take to the ski slopes, mountain trails, and golf courses despite their physical limitations.

THE BOTTOM LINE ON STEP 2
Get Up and Get Moving

- ▶ If you've been sedentary and have had diabetes for 10 years or more, you may want to see your doctor before starting any higher-intensity exercise.
- ▶ Adding more steps in every day is the easiest and surest way to start moving more.

- ► Consider getting a pedometer to monitor your daily steps and to act as a motivator.
- ► Every bit of movement you do during the day—whether spontaneous or planned—counts.
- ► Even standing, talking, and fidgeting use up extra calories and can make a difference in your body weight and insulin sensitivity.
- ► Cardio, strength, toning, and flexibility exercises can give you additional health benefits.
- ► You can exercise safely and effectively with most diabetic complications and other health limitations, including excess body weight, arthritis, and orthopedic problems.
- ► Non-weight-bearing exercises, such as aquatic activities, stationary cycling, and armchair exercises, are a viable way for almost everyone to become physically active.
- ► Having diabetes should be your main reason for becoming more physically active, not an excuse to forego all activity.

Now that you know all about what exercise can do for you and which precautions you should take for your particular needs, keep reading to learn how to train correctly and effectively to get the most out of any physical activity. Remember that becoming physically fit is the only guaranteed way to live well with (or without) diabetes.

DIABETES FITNESS PLAN STEP 2
in a Nutshell

REGARDLESS OF your current physical condition, there are myriad easy and effective ways to start moving more to make the undeniable benefits of increased physical activity on your diabetes control and general health yours to keep for the rest of your life.

STEP 3

Become Even More Fit

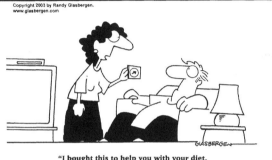

"I bought this to help you with your diet.
It's a compass that always points to exercise equipment."

AFTER HAVING FOCUSED on weight loss as your primary goal all these years, you may be having trouble switching gears and focusing on becoming more active and fit instead. However, you now know that you can become healthy without losing all (or even any) of your excess weight. And if you do manage to lose some weight, you'll only be likely to keep it off if you're regularly physically active. So, your new goal should be to stop worrying about your weight and instead become as physically active as possible each and every day to maximize your caloric expenditure and BG use—and you don't necessarily have to join the nearest gym to do so. Just take the stairs instead of the elevator; park your car at the far end of the lot; walk in place during TV commercials; use fewer labor-saving devices; and take the dog out for a walk as part of your daily routine.

However, while simply moving more is extremely beneficial to your overall health and diabetes control, you should also focus on maximizing your physical activities. Even for myself, I find that if I don't occasionally include a harder workout in my weekly routine, my insulin sensitivity starts to backslide. Thus, the third step on your way to diabetes fitness is to optimize your fitness and insulin action from the activities you do by getting the most that you possibly can out of each and every one of them. For example, walking is good to get you started moving, but you can further enhance your fitness by varying your walking speed and distance. You'll learn lots of "tricks" to help you optimize every type of activity in this fitness step, along with proper techniques for exercises, appropriate stretches, easy resistance exercises that you can do at home or away, and methods for preventing and dealing with the inevitable occasional muscle soreness or athletic injury.

In the remainder of this step, you will find some sample workouts and learn many more helpful pointers. My goal is to help you maximize your fitness by working specifically on your endurance, strength, flexibility, and body "core."

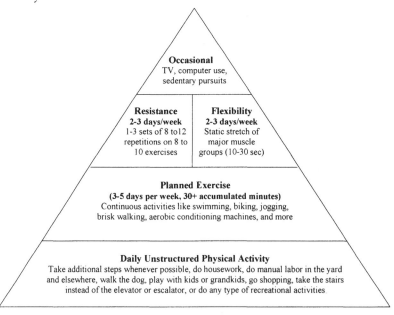

Occasional
TV, computer use,
sedentary pursuits

Resistance
2-3 days/week
1-3 sets of 8 to12
repetitions on 8 to
10 exercises

Flexibility
2-3 days/week
Static stretch of
major muscle
groups (10-30 sec)

Planned Exercise
(3-5 days per week, 30+ accumulated minutes)
Continuous activities like swimming, biking, jogging,
brisk walking, aerobic conditioning machines, and more

Daily Unstructured Physical Activity
Take additional steps whenever possible, do housework, do manual labor in the yard
and elsewhere, walk the dog, play with kids or grandkids, go shopping, take the stairs
instead of the elevator or escalator, or do any type of recreational activities.

A physical activity pyramid is a good starting place

To enhance your basic understanding of the various components of an overall plan for optimal fitness, you can use a physical activity "pyramid" (similar in concept to older versions of the food guide pyramid) to give general recommendations for appropriate daily physical activity for adults and older teens. The base of this pyramid recommends that you fill each day with unstructured activities simply by being as active as possible. It includes activities such as walking, doing housework, gardening, and the like. The next level recommends a minimum of 30 minutes of aerobic exercise or recreational sports three to five days per week, including more structured activities such as cycling or swimming. Both strength and flexibility activities are listed in the two to three days per week range. Finally, cutting down on all sedentary pursuits, including TV watching, computer and video games, and sitting for more than 30 minutes at a time for any reason is strongly recommended.

While this pyramid is a good place to start, it's vitally important that you structure your own exercise plan. If you don't tailor it to your individual needs and desires, it will be doomed to fail. Once you have completed step 2 and are moving more, you will benefit further from including more structured aerobic activities, such as planned walking or using a treadmill, stationary cycle, rower, or other aerobic workout machine on a regular basis. Increasing your endurance is not as hard as you might think, but you'll need to start out very conservatively in order to allow your body time to adapt to your new activity. Move in the direction of exercising a minimum of three days a week for 20 to 30 minutes a day (for a minimum of 10 minutes at a time), and then gradually work up to 45 to 60 minutes per day and/or five days per week for optimal fitness gains.

Include warmups and cool-downs in every workout session

It's vitally important that you warm your body up before you begin any more intense workout in order to get your blood pumping and to prepare yourself mentally for activity. A **warmup** serves to raise your core body temperature, which also means that the oxygen supply to your muscles is increased, your muscles are more flexible, and your heart, lungs, and other organs are prepared for a period of activity. A short period (at least five minutes) of low-intensity aerobic activity, such as marching in place or slow walking, is a good way to warm up your whole body. Your muscles and joints should ideally be stretched after your body temperature has been raised and blood flow to your muscles has been increased through easy aerobic activity of some type. Slow, gentle stretches then help to warm the muscles up further and relieve any tension.

A **cool-down** serves an equally important purpose: to minimize post-exercise muscle fatigue, soreness, and stiffness. The cool-down period is similar to the warmup and should consist of 5 to 10 minutes (the harder the exercise, the longer the cool-down) of low-intensity exercise, such as slow walking again, at the end of your activity. During this time your heart rate returns to normal, metabolic by-products such as excess lactic acid are removed from the muscles, and your body temperature goes down. Pain felt in muscles immediately after exercise is usually the result of residual lactic acid produced during the activity. Cooling down allows your body to remove such by-products of exercise faster, reducing any postexercise discomfort and stiffness. After your cool-down, you should gently stretch out any tense muscles to reduce cramping or tightness and improve flexibility.

Training tips to get the most out of your aerobic workouts

Like most people, you may find that planned workouts are much harder to fit into your daily routine. Studies have shown that people are more likely to consistently accumulate the recommended amounts of physical activity during the day by increasing their unstructured activities rather than by following a formal exercise program, primarily due to time constraints or a perceived lack of time for structured sessions. Also, you'll need a higher level of motivation to continue participating in preplanned exercise over time; rates of continued participation are notoriously abysmal. At worst, if you can't manage to do regular workouts consistently, it pays to emphasize the unstructured ones on a daily basis. Still, structured aerobic workouts undeniably have their benefits and I highly recommend them for achieving overall good health and a higher level of physical fitness.

Easy Ways to Add in Structured Aerobic Exercise

▶ Participate in after-work team activities such as soccer, softball, or basketball; take dance classes; or sign up for any other activity that you enjoy.
▶ Get involved in community physical activities, such as fun runs and health walks that require you to train for them.
▶ Find the nearest tennis courts and start playing regularly (take lessons, if needed), or find the nearest basketball court and start using it regularly.

► Go for walks whenever possible on weekends or in the evenings, and include the whole family, neighbors, or friends.

► Instead of driving, walk, run, or bike wherever you need to go whenever possible.

► Dust off your home exercise equipment, particularly a stationary bike, treadmill, rebounder, or rower, and start using it while watching your favorite TV shows or listening to music.

► If you join a gym or other exercise facility, find one that is convenient to your home or work to increase the likelihood that you will actually use it regularly.

► Set aside 15 to 20 minutes a day to walk, run, or step in place with your significant other or the whole family while you talk about your day.

By definition, an **aerobic** activity is one that uses your large muscles rhythmically and continuously for more than two minutes at a time. Accordingly, all of the more traditional exercises (i.e., walking, jogging, cycling, swimming, aerobic dance, and more) qualify, but so do some of the newer ones, such as in-line skating, aquatic exercise classes, "hip hop dancing" classes, and some segments of Pilates workouts, just to name a few. An alternative to the more traditional forms of aerobic exercise is participation in more recreational (but planned) after-work or weekend activities such as soccer, softball, or basketball, or ballroom dancing. The current recommendation for everyone is a minimum of three to five days per week of aerobic exercise done for 30 to 60 minutes—either continuously or cumulatively, as long as it occurs in bouts of 10 minutes or longer.

Interval training. Now that you know the basics of aerobic training, it's time to learn some tricks to get even more fit while doing these activities. For starters, during any activity, simply increase the intensity of your exercise for short periods of time (so-called interval training) to gain more from it. For example, if you are out walking, speed up slightly for a short distance (such as between two light poles or mailboxes) before slowing back down to your original pace. During the course of your walk, continue to include these short, faster intervals occasionally, and, as you are able to, lengthen these intervals so that they last two to five minutes at a time. Not only will you become more fit and use up extra calories doing so, but you also will likely feel more tired when you finish your walk (which is actually a good thing). Over the course of several weeks, you may even find that your general walking speed has increased due to the extra conditioning from your interspersed bouts of faster walking.

By way of example, when unfit men and women in their 30s and 40s trained just twice a week doing only three to four minutes of aerobic exercise at an intensity of 70 to 80 percent of their maximal heart rate (i.e., short, intense exercise), preceded and followed by three-minute warmup and cool-down periods, they increased their maximal aerobic capacity by over 13 percent in twelve weeks—and most people can't increase their maximal capacity by more than 25 percent total, no matter how much or how long they train. Almost unbelievably, the participants in this study experienced major gains in their aerobic capacity by doing only six to eight minutes of harder exercise a week.

Perhaps studies like these explain the sudden interest in the ROM Time Machine, an exercise machine available in specialized gyms that you work on for only four minutes at a time, but at a near-maximal pace. It's definitely not going to get you as fit as longer sessions of aerobic exercise, and it certainly won't prepare you to run a marathon, but it has its benefits. The same intensity principle applies to almost every kind of exercise you do, from walking to cycling to gardening. In fact, even competitive athletes generally plateau at a certain level unless they do some version of this heavier "interval" training from time to time.

TIP

16

NO MATTER YOUR WEIGHT

YOU MAY be able to make major gains in your aerobic fitness level just by adding in as little as six to eight minutes of harder exercise a week to your current workouts. Try interspersing short periods of faster walking or harder intervals into whatever exercise you are doing for optimal gains.

An alternate way to do intervals is just to vary the way that you are doing an activity. With walking, this could involve alternately taking longer and then shorter strides for short periods of time. This method may not be as effective in terms of aerobic fitness as doing harder training, but it may encourage you to use a wider range of motion, which can help enhance the flexibility of your joints (e.g., hip, knee, and ankle joints for walking). Adding in arm movement, such as pumping your arms in an exaggerated manner while walking, can also benefit both your aerobic fitness and your upper-body flexibility.

Tips for Optimizing Your Endurance Training

▶ Become more active all day in unstructured ways to build your overall endurance.

▶ Incorporate faster intervals into any activity that you do.

▶ Plan workouts of varying intensities or hard and easy days to maximize results.

▶ Incorporate at least one long day of exercise a week to build greater endurance.

▶ To maximize your insulin action, aim to spend a greater total time being active rather than worrying about your workout intensity.

▶ If you can only manage to fit in short workouts, try to work out harder during that time to gain or preserve fitness.

▶ Emphasize the fullest range of motion possible around your joints during all activities.

▶ Participate in a variety of activities to gain the benefits of cross training and to keep your interest high and your injuries few.

▶ Include at least one day of rest into your weekly schedule, but ideally avoid taking off more than two days in a row.

Hard and easy days. Another means of enhancing overall fitness and insulin sensitivity is to incorporate workouts of varying intensities into your weekly routine. Actually, it is better for a number of physiological (as well as psychological) reasons to alternate easy and hard workouts. Almost all seasoned athletes vary their training in this manner, and for good reason: in order for your body to fully recover from intense workouts, it needs adequate rest, which includes not just proper amounts of sleep (seven to eight hours a night for most adults), but also enough time between workouts to fully rebuild muscle, restore glycogen, and recuperate. Easy workouts do not cause the same level of glycogen depletion and muscle damage as harder ones and, thus, constitute a form of rest in themselves. However, with regard to maximizing your insulin action, the total amount of exercise you do is still more important than the workout's intensity.

TIP
17

NO MATTER YOUR WEIGHT

DOING CLOSE to three hours (170 minutes) of exercise per week at any intensity improves insulin sensitivity more than if you accumulate only two hours of activity (115 minutes) weekly, regardless of the intensity of your exercise. The length of your physical activities, therefore, appears to be more important for your BG control than their intensity.

By alternating workout intensities (mild, moderate, and heavy), your body will get both the enhanced fitness and strength benefits of hard workouts and the healing effects of greater recuperative time between intense workouts. Doing so also prevents **overuse syndrome**, which results from overstressing your body with repeated heavy workouts and manifests itself as frequent colds, chronic tiredness, and joint and muscle injuries. A day of rest at least once a week is vitally important, even if on that day you do a different activity or something low-intensity. But don't let more than two days elapse between workouts if you want to maintain your heightened insulin action.

When you do become more fit, your workouts may feel easier (at least most of the time). At that point, if you want to continue making fitness gains, you can make your workouts either longer or more intense. For example, if you've been walking 30 minutes and you're so fit now that your walk hardly even makes you feel tired or winded, either increase your walking time to 45 minutes or walk at a faster pace to maximize your fitness and insulin sensitivity gains. If for some reason you have to cut back the total amount of time that you are training, try to maintain a higher workout intensity, as working out harder (even if for much less time) will actually preserve your level of fitness more effectively than doing longer, easier workouts. Alternately, you can include intermittent short bouts of harder intensity throughout your workout.

Distance training. To improve your overall fitness (endurance) base, you can also try **LSD training**. Perhaps when you see the acronym "LSD," you're thrown back to the 1960s and hallucinogenic recreational drugs. Time to modernize your thinking. Nowadays, LSD refers to "long, slow distance training," which serves to generally build up your endurance. If you do only short bouts of activity—such as 10 minutes at a time—do you really think that your body will be able to withstand a one-hour walk without leaving you feeling excessively tired? Not likely. It is for this reason that people training to run longer races or marathons usually do at least one long run a week, often on the weekend when they have more time. Your endurance will likewise be vastly enhanced if you exercise longer than normal at least once a week; doing so will help you build up your endurance base, which will in turn make every other activity a little easier to do—and you won't tire out as quickly.

Cross training. Another simple way to become more fit, believe it or not, is simply to do a wide variety of activities. For example, you could walk for 30 to 60 minutes on Monday, Wednesday, and Friday, but swim on Tuesday and take dance classes on Saturday. Cross training is really the key to avoiding overuse injuries, keeping your exercise fresh and fun, and achieving maximal fitness.

In terms of controlling glycemia, this approach is also very effective. Each activity uses muscles differently, recruiting either different muscles altogether or the same ones in different patterns, which results in a wider use of your whole body. Since you do each activity less frequently when you vary them, though, you will likely not experience as pronounced of a training effect, meaning that you will use more of your BG during activities that you do less frequently—which is not necessarily bad if you're using your workouts to help lower your BG levels.

Monitoring exercise intensity. If you are motivated by checking your heart rate during exercise, consult Appendix B for precalculated **target heart rates** recommended for optimal endurance gains. You can easily measure your own heart rate by placing two fingers (not your thumb) on your radial artery (found on your wrist right below the base of your thumb) or on your carotid artery (found on the side of your neck about two inches forward and three inches down from your earlobe under your jaw). Count the total number of beats that you feel in 15 seconds, then multiply by four to equal your minute heart rate. Alternately, you can invest in an inexpensive heart-rate monitor that you can wear to measure your heart rate for you.

You really won't need a heart-rate monitor to know when you're working out harder than you need to. Just use the **Talk Test** (i.e., you shouldn't be breathing too heavily to talk to someone else while exercising) when doing any type of interval or intense training to keep from training harder than necessary for your fitness and BG goals. Few additional fitness gains will result from working out so hard that you feel short of breath or extremely fatigued, since the amount of time you can maintain such a workout intensity is severely limited. Working out too hard is also, for many people, a big deterrent to maintaining their aerobic exercise regimens, which is another reason to not make it too hard for yourself.

TIP
18

NO MATTER YOUR WEIGHT

INSTEAD OF measuring your heart rate, you can use the Talk Test to easily tell when you may be working out harder than you need to. To "pass" the test, you should not be breathing so heavily during an activity that you're not able to carry on a conversation with someone else at the same time without gasping for breath. Exercising too intensely increases your risk of injury, as well as the chance that you will not continue to exercise regularly.

Lastly, forget about the "fat burning" and the "cardio training" heart-rate ranges that you find on many workout machines. As long as you're working hard enough to expend extra calories (which is pretty much by doing any activity at all), then you're meeting your primary goal; the type of fuel you're using during exercise doesn't matter. The "fat burning" ranges are irrelevant, because your body uses more carbohydrate than fat during almost all intensities of exercise. Besides, during all the time that you're recovering from your exercise (i.e., the twenty-three or more hours a day you aren't exercising), your body is mainly metabolizing fat, so it really makes no difference what type of fuel mix your body uses during the hour or less that you're active. If you want to optimize your aerobic fitness gains and be in the "cardio training" ranges, though, aim for at least the bottom end of the heart-rate range in Appendix B, which is equivalent to 50 percent of your maximal capacity with your resting heart rate taken into account.

Resistance exercises: How and where to do them

Sets, reps, and other training basics. Some examples of traditional strength training exercises are biceps curls, abdominal crunches, bench presses, leg presses, lunges, and calf raises (more on these exercises to come). The current recommendation is to resistance train two to three nonconsecutive days per week and include all the major muscle groups of your body. If you are a novice at resistance work, you can start out with lighter weights or more flexible resistance bands that enable you to complete one to two **sets** of 12 to 15 **repetitions** (a.k.a. reps) on each exercise.

TIP
19

NO MATTER YOUR WEIGHT

WHEN TWO to three sets of 15 reps are easy for you to do (that is, you feel like you could do even more), make your resistance workouts progressive by adding some weight or resistance to each exercise and dropping the number of reps you are doing in each set back to no more than 12 to avoid reaching a plateau in your strength gains.

When you have completed this elementary stage of your weight program for six to eight weeks, you will be able to handle heavier weights and perform fewer reps per set. Ideally, your goal is to drop the number of reps that you can actually complete down into the range of 8 to 12 reps per set for optimal strength gains (and besides, aiming for an even 10 reps is easy to remember). While focusing on more reps using lower weights increases **muscular endurance** more effectively, lifting a greater resistance for fewer reps generally produces more **overload** on the muscle fibers and greater gains in **muscular strength**; consequently, you'll recruit the faster fibers during the work, all of your muscle fibers will increase in size faster, and you'll add more muscle mass. As a result, your muscles will then use more calories even at rest, your resting **metabolism** will increase, and your insulin sensitivity will improve. Alternately, when doing more than one set per exercise, you can increase the weight or resistance on each successive set, slightly decreasing the number of reps each time the load increases (for example, from 15 reps on the first down to 10 on the second, harder set).

How much versus how often. Having said all that, I now have to backtrack and say that, according to the latest research on older individuals, it appears to be far less important to focus on how much weight you lift than to simply make sure that you are lifting some. For instance, a study on postmenopausal women showed that both high-load (heavy weights, fewer reps) and high-repetition (lighter weights, more reps) resistance training were effective in increasing muscular strength and size, indicating that even easy resistance training is beneficial for older women. Likewise, muscular endurance, strength, and stair-climbing time improved in adults aged 60 to 83 doing only one set of 12 resistance exercises at either 50 percent of their 1-rep max (the maximum amount they can lift one time) for 13 reps or 80 percent of **1-rep max** for 8 reps, which the participants did thrice weekly for 24 weeks.

Basically, then, you can choose either training regimen—lighter weights and more reps or heavier weights and fewer reps—and likely experience similar gains. You may even decide to vary easy days, where you do more reps with lighter weights, and hard days, when you lift heavier weights fewer times, depending on how motivated you feel on a given day and how much time you have to train. The only resistance training principles you absolutely need to follow are (1) to work a particular area of your body (i.e., upper body) no more frequently than every other day, and (2) to equally train muscles with opposite actions on a joint, such as the biceps and triceps muscles of your upper arm or the quadriceps and hamstring muscles of your thigh.

Resistance Training Dos and Don'ts

Do:

- Do resistance training that includes exercises using all parts of your body (upper and lower body, abdominal area, and lower back) two to three nonconsecutive days per week
- During each workout session, start with exercises that use multiple muscle groups first (e.g., thighs), and then isolate smaller muscle groups with additional exercises
- Train opposing muscle groups (such as biceps and triceps) equally to avoid injuries
- Do at least one set per exercise, preferably doing 8 to 12 repetitions to complete exhaustion
- Exhale fully as you work against or lift the resistance and inhale during the return to the starting position
- Take two to three minutes of rest between multiple sets on the same exercise
- Use as full a range of motion as possible around each joint during all exercises
- Allow at least 48 hours to recuperate between training on specific parts of your body (i.e., upper body, lower body, etc.)
- Stretch during and/or after resistance training workouts for greater strength gains
- During the first few weeks of training, focus on good body mechanics and technique, and then add on more weight or resistance—slowly

▶ Keep your torso and spine straight during all exercises (except abs and lower-back work)

▶ Consider finding a workout facility or gym that has either resistance training machines or free weights that you can use to push yourself with once your strength increases

Don't:

▶ Lock your knees when your legs are supporting the weight (or your elbows during upper-body work)

▶ Pick up any weights off the floor by bending over with straight legs

▶ Fatigue your abdominal ("core") muscles before completing other exercises, particularly when using free weights or resistance bands (as opposed to weight machines)

▶ Work the same muscle groups two consecutive days

▶ Hold your breath while doing resistance work

▶ Unduly twist your back or spine when doing any resistance work

▶ Do sit-ups with your back straight (rather than curling forward)

▶ Sacrifice your form just to add more weight, resistance, or repetitions

▶ Continue with an exercise if you feel a sharp or immediate pain in any joint or muscle

▶ Worry about how much you are lifting; instead, focus on making sure that you do resistance training at least once a week

Getting more out of resistance training in less time. Not surprisingly, doing multiple sets (two or more) on each exercise results in greater strength gains than doing just one. Nevertheless, as long as you do a minimum of one set, you will gain strength. Personally, I just can't seem to find the time to spend the hours in a weight room that are required to do multiple sets on every exercise I need to do. As a result, nowadays my workouts are more focused on gaining the most I can from doing less, which means that I do only one set on each exercise, but I make sure to completely wear out my working muscles by the time I complete my targeted number of reps (usually 8 to 12) for that single set.

Whether you do one set or more, the real key to maximizing your strength gains is to use enough weight or resistance for the number of reps you do on each exercise to fully fatigue your muscles. For a range of 8 to 12 reps, this workload will likely be 70 to 90 percent of your 1-rep max. No matter how much you lift, though, your goal is to be completely fatigued within the range of reps you have chosen. For example, you should be able to complete at least 8 but no more than 12 reps for a chosen range of 8 to 12 reps. Even if you can only fit in one set on each exercise once a week, you will still experience some strength gains, particularly if you max yourself out on each and every set.

Interestingly, more strength is gained both when you emphasize a full range of motion around each joint and when you do stretching along with the resistance exercises. To incorporate a full range of movement, you may have to use a lighter load to accomplish the same number of reps, but the overall results are better. As far as stretching exercised muscles, anytime you start to feel tight during your workout, stop and stretch out that muscle. In terms of strength gains, though, it doesn't matter whether you stretch between exercises or all at once at the end of your workout.

Important tips for preventing injuries. Muscle tears and pulls or joint injuries are mostly avoidable if you incorporate proper weight-lifting techniques and stretching, and if you lift more slowly, without excess speed or bouncing movements. Also, the range of motion you use should be limited to pain-free arcs. Equally important to injury prevention is giving your body adequate rest periods between sets in a workout (at least two to three minutes between each set), as well as adequate rest (a minimum of 48 hours) between resistance-training workouts using the same muscle groups.

Emphasize working larger groups of muscles first, before you isolate and work individual muscles within those groups (e.g., do leg-press exercises to train all of your lower-body musculature together before doing exercises to isolate the quadriceps on the front of your thigh). It also helps to vary the order of your exercises, so that you don't work the same muscles consecutively without at least a small break in between to allow your first energy system (phosphagens) to fully replenish between sets (which it does in two to three minutes). Plan on doing abdominal exercises last—at the very end of your workout—so that you haven't fatigued these muscles before you have to rely on them to maintain your posture during other exercises.

Finally, a word about the proper way to breathe during resistance exercises. In general, when you are lifting a weight or working muscles against a resistance or gravity, exhale through your mouth as you are performing the work. This portion of the exercise (the **concentric** portion) is usually done during a count of two ("one, two"). When you are returning to the starting position in the direction that gravity is pulling the weight (i.e., doing **eccentric** work that causes a greater overload on the muscle and enhanced strength gains), silently count to four ("one, two, three, four") to emphasize the eccentric portion of the lift, and inhale throughout the motion.

TIP
20

NO MATTER YOUR WEIGHT

NEVER—AND I repeat, never—hold your breath while you are doing any resistance training work. Doing so may cause an excessive rise in your blood pressure and lead to a stroke, heart attack, or other cardiovascular event.

Training equipment and location. You can purchase inexpensive resistance training bands, such as Dyna-Bands or other rubber tubing, from almost any sporting-goods store, certain superstores, chain drugstores, and online; resistance bands sold for Pilates and other workouts can be used as well. Many varieties allow you to progress your training by using bands of varying resistance (usually color-coded so that you can tell which ones offer easy, medium, or hard resistance). Some bands are like wide strips of a flexible, rubbery substance that you can grip with your hands or tie. (If you tie the band during certain exercises, use a simple bow or a square knot.) Other bands look more like thin rubber tubing and may come with attached handles, and some are like big rubber bands or figure eights. You can make any of these bands work for you, so buy whichever ones you feel most comfortable with.

If you would prefer to use more traditional dumbbells during exercises, pick up an inexpensive set of small ones. If you're just starting out, get a set that ranges in weight from 1 to 10 pounds, or possibly a smaller range, like 1-pound, 3-pound, and 5-pound weights to start with. If you're strong enough that small weights are extremely easy to lift, you may want to either invest in a costlier set of heavier weights or consider joining the nearest gym or workout facility to have access to heavier loads and resistance machines. If you would rather not invest in any weights, you can get creative using household items of varying weights that you can easily grasp in your hands (some examples follow).

Some basic resistance-training exercises that you can do using hand weights and/or resistance bands are illustrated in the following sections. Both upper-body and lower-body exercises are included, but lower-back and abdominal-strength exercises—which are equally important—are not given until you reach the strong "core" section later in this step. Some resistance exercises using household items are included as well, and you can also fit in some "unstructured" weight training by lifting items around the house (including kids and grandkids).

As for unstructured or resistance work using household items, however, be forewarned that a recent study showed that for older adults with type 2 diabetes, home-based resistance training was not effective for maintaining normal **glycemia**, although improvements in muscle strength and muscle mass were equivalent to those achieved in a gym. In that study, the reduced adherence to regular training and the 52 percent reduction in the intensity of training at home (due to people not having access to weight-training machines) likely lessened the impact of the home-based resistance work on BG, which is most reflective of how much muscle glycogen you use during workout sessions. If you use lighter weights, you will use up less glycogen and, accordingly, have a smaller impact on your insulin action and your BG. Lighter training also recruits and trains fewer muscle fibers, resulting in a smaller increase in muscle mass following training. Still, if you have to choose between an easier, home-based program and no training at all, stick with whatever you can manage to do at home.

TIP
21

NO MATTER YOUR WEIGHT

TRAINING BY doing routine functional tasks actually improves your ability to do such work more effectively than doing less specific resistance training. So, it's entirely possible for you to gain benefits and remain independent by doing your "unstructured" resistance tasks or resistance training at home.

Muscle identification. In figuring out which training exercises to do, it's helpful to have a basic understanding of which muscle(s) are being used for each activity, including the muscle names and their general location (i.e., shoulder, upper arm, thigh, etc.). In the upper body, you have muscles that include the shoulder deltoids (front, medial, and back portions), pectoralis major and minor (the pectorals, or "pecs") on the front of your chest, upper back and neck muscles (latissimus dorsi or "lats," trapezius, and rhomboids), and biceps (front) and triceps (back) of your upper arm. Your main lower-body muscles include the quadriceps ("quads") and hamstrings on the front and back of your thighs, respectively, adductors (inner thigh), gluteus muscles ("gluts" or buttocks), and calf muscles (gastrocnemius and soleus). Finally, your main abdominal muscle directly in front and down the center is the rectus abdominus, but all of the stomach muscles together (including the internal and external obliques on your sides) are collectively called "abdominal muscles," or "abs."

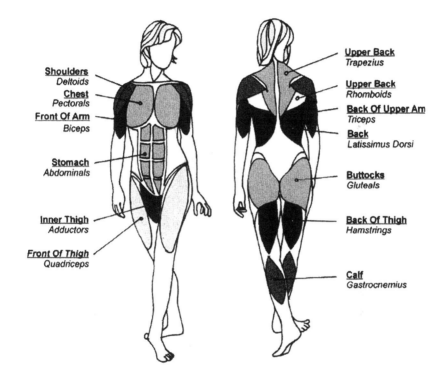

Shoulders
Deltoids

Chest
Pectorals

Front Of Arm
Biceps

Stomach
Abdominals

Inner Thigh
Adductors

Front Of Thigh
Quadriceps

Upper Back
Trapezius

Upper Back
Rhomboids

Back Of Upper Arm
Triceps

Back
Latissimus Dorsi

Buttocks
Gluteals

Back Of Thigh
Hamstrings

Calf
Gastrocnemius

Refer to the muscle chart to learn the muscles and muscle groups most often targeted during training. The resistance exercises that follow list the main muscle groups involved in each one, thus enabling you to work on different muscles or muscle groups and include all of the main ones in the exercises that you choose to do. Having a basic understanding of your own musculature also allows you to choose exercises that emphasize working multiple muscles or muscle groups first, followed by isolated muscles (for example, doing chest-press exercises first before isolating the front of the arm with biceps curls), which is the recommended progression of exercises to maximize your gains and avoid injuries.

Upper-Body Exercises

1

CHEST PRESS

Equipment: dumbbells or resistance band, exercise mat (optional)
Main muscles worked: deltoid (front section), pecs, triceps

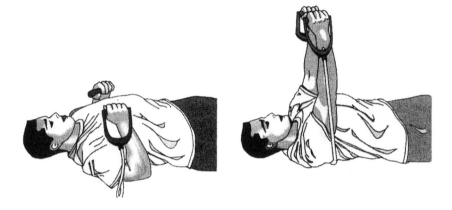

Directions:

Lie down on your back holding a dumbbell in each hand right above your chest with your elbows bent; if you're using a resistance band, position the band underneath your shoulders and grab onto it with your hands.

Push both arms up in the air until they are almost straight, shoulder-width apart, and hold this position for several seconds.

Bring your arms back down to your sides until your elbows touch the mat, allowing the dumbbells (or resistance band) to come back to the starting position.

2
SHOULDER PRESS

Equipment: dumbbells or resistance band, upright chair or bench
Main muscles worked: deltoids (anterior and middle portion), trapezius, triceps

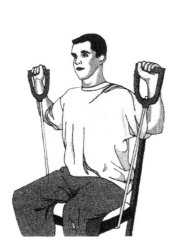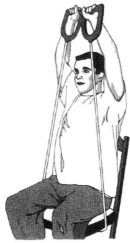

Directions:

In a sitting position, hold the dumbbells right above your shoulders with bent elbows, or, if using a resistance band, sit on it and hold the band on either side at shoulder height.

Keep your abdominal muscles tight and your torso straight.

Push up until your arms are almost straight and the dumbbells or your hands come close to meeting in the middle above your head.

Slowly return to the starting position.

3

LATERAL RAISE

Equipment: dumbbells or resistance band, bench or armless chair
Main muscles worked: deltoid (middle and back sections), trapezius

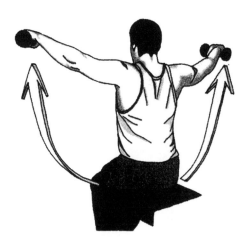

Directions:

Sit with your back straight and the dumbbells in your hands at your sides or the resistance band underneath your bottom.

If using the resistance band, grasp one end of it in each hand and clench your fists with your knuckles facing upward.

Lift the dumbbells (or pull the resistance band up and straight out to the side) until both arms are level with your shoulders, keeping your elbows slightly bent.

Hold this position for a few seconds before slowly returning to the starting position.

During this exercise, relax your neck and try not to hunch your shoulders to ensure that your shoulder and neck muscles are doing the work (and not your arms).

4

MODIFIED PUSH-UPS

Equipment: resistance band, exercise mat (optional)
Main muscles worked: pecs, deltoids (anterior portion), triceps

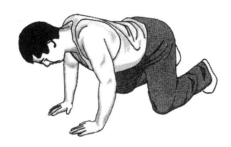

Directions:

Get on your hands and knees on the floor or mat.

If using a band for extra resistance, position it across your back and hold one end of it in each hand so that it is somewhat tight when your elbows are straight.

Place your hands shoulder-width apart on the mat.

Tighten your abdominal muscles to straighten your lower back and lower yourself (from your knees, not your feet) down toward the mat as far as you can without touching it.

Push yourself back up until your arms are extended, but without locking your elbows.

If this exercise is too hard, stand facing a wall and place your arms on it at shoulder height and your feet about a foot away; then, do your push-ups off the wall (with or without a resistance band).

5

DOUBLE-ARM ROW

Equipment: dumbbells or resistance band, exercise mat (optional)
Main muscles worked: deltoids (back portion), lats, rhomboids, biceps

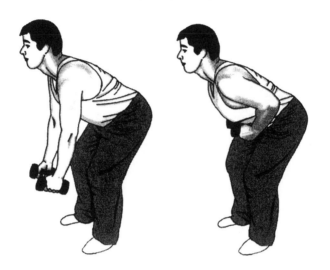

Directions:

Stand with your feet in line with your hips with a dumbbell in each
hand.

If using a resistance band, position it underneath your feet and hold the
band with both hands at your sides.

With your knees slightly bent, bend your upper body forward from the
hips about 70 degrees.

Straighten your arms so that your palms face each other.

Pull the dumbbells or resistance band in toward your waist so that your
elbows move up past your hips, but with your upper arms staying
close to your sides.

Alternately, sit with your legs out in front of you (knees slightly bent)
and the resistance band wrapped around the soles of both feet; then,
keeping your torso straight, pull your arms straight back, keeping your
arms by your sides during the movement.

6

LAT PULL-DOWN

Equipment: resistance band, chair or bench
Main muscles worked: lats, biceps

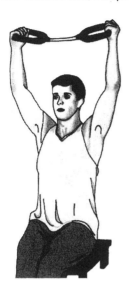 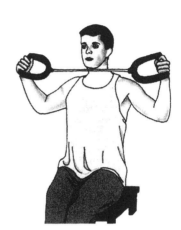

Directions:

Sit with your back straight and hold both ends of the resistance band, one in each hand.

Still grasping the band, fully extend your arms above your head.

With your arms still extended, stretch the band so that both hands go out to the sides slightly wider than your shoulders, and hold this position for a few seconds.

Pull the stretched band down toward your chin, pulling out on the band by bending at the elbow to stretch it more.

Squeeze your shoulder blades together and feel the muscles in your back, shoulders, and arms contract.

Hold this position for a few seconds and then extend your arms back up above your head, allowing the band to relax.

7

BICEPS CURLS

Equipment: dumbbells or resistance band, upright chair or bench
Main muscles worked: biceps

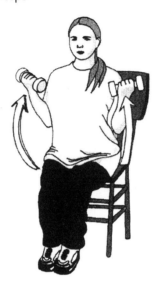

Directions:

Sit down holding the dumbbells, and drop both arms to your sides so that your elbows are in line with your hips with your palms facing forward.

Bring your knees and feet together, keeping your stomach muscles tight to support your lower back.

Lift the dumbbells, bending your elbows while keeping your upper arms stationary at your sides until the dumbbells almost touch your chest.

Slowly return the dumbbells to the starting position.

Alternately, do one arm at a time by supporting the elbow of the arm holding the dumbbell against the inside of your knee on the same side.

With resistance bands, secure one end of the band under your right foot and grasp the other end in your right hand, palm face up, and complete the same movement, keeping your upper arm close to your torso at all times; switch sides to work the left arm.

8

TRICEPS CURLS

Equipment: dumbbells or resistance band, upright chair or bench
Main muscles worked: triceps

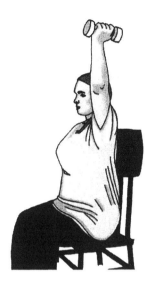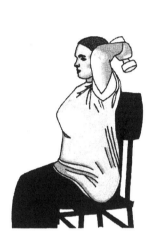

Directions:

Sit on the bench or chair holding one dumbbell in your lap with both hands.

Lift the dumbbell straight up until your arms are straight and the dumbbell is directly overhead.

Bend your arms at the elbows only and lower the dumbbell behind your head.

Keep your stomach muscles tight throughout the movement to support your lower back and keep it straight.

Lift the dumbbell straight overhead again by straightening your arms at the elbow to return to the starting position.

If using a resistance band, hold it in your right hand while you raise your right arm with bent elbow, and drop the band straight down behind your back on the right side; then grab the other end in your left hand by reaching behind across the small of your back. Alternately straighten and bend at the elbow (with your upper arm still raised at the shoulder), and then switch the positioning of your arms to work the left side.

At-Home Versions of Upper-Body Exercises

YOU SHOULD be able to easily add in resistance training without joining a gym or even buying expensive equipment for your home. If you'd rather not have to get some resistance bands or small dumbbells, try the following easy versions of the same upper-body work detailed above that you can do using items you already have around the house.

Flour chest-press (upper-body exercise 1): Do the chest press using 5- or 10-pound bags of flour (or a lighter bag of cornmeal to start) held in both hands.

Spaghetti-sauce shoulder press (upper-body exercise 2): Try the shoulder press holding a full jar of spaghetti sauce in each hand (use larger or heavier jars as you are able).

Bottled water lateral raise (upper-body exercise 3): Do your lateral raises holding water bottles of varying weights (12-ounce, 20-ounce, 1-liter, or 2-liter sizes).

Dictionary modified push-ups (upper-body exercise 4): Vary your modified push-ups by having someone place a dictionary (or a 5-pound bag of flour) in the middle of your back after you assume the starting position on the floor.

Broom double-arm row (upper-body exercise 5): Do a variation of double-arm rowing while holding a broom or mop; for more weight, tie milk jugs or bottles on each end filled with varying amounts of water.

Mop pull-down (upper-body exercise 6): Try a variation of lat pull-downs by holding a mop or broom with your hands as far apart as is comfortable; to add more weight, follow instructions for double-arm row (above).

Soup-can biceps and triceps curls (upper-body exercises 7 and 8): Do your biceps and triceps curls holding a soup can in your hand (or try larger cans, jars, or water bottles for more weight).

Lower-Body Exercises

1

ONE-LEG PRESS

Equipment: resistance band, exercise mat (optional)
Main muscles worked: quads, gluts, calves

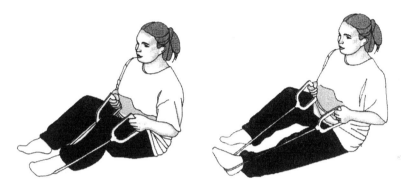

Directions:

Sit on the floor with your legs out in front of you, knees slightly bent.

Hold one end of the resistance band in each hand and place it around
the sole of your right foot with your right knee fully bent.

Straighten your right leg (without locking your knee) while pulling on
both sides of the resistance band.

Continue to pull against the resistance band as you return your knee to
the bent position.

Repeat the exercise with your left leg.

Alternately, tie the resistance band in a circle around the leg of a chair,
then sit on the chair, place the sole of your foot inside the other end
of the band, and straighten your leg almost fully out.

2

SQUATS

Equipment: dumbbells or resistance band
Main muscles worked: quads, hamstrings, gluts, calves

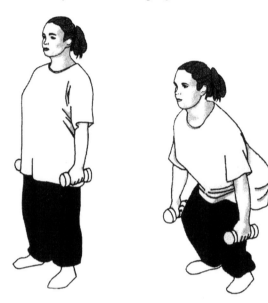

Directions:

Stand with a dumbbell in each hand and your feet shoulder-width apart, with your toes pointing slightly out to the side.

If you're using a resistance band, tie both ends of your band onto a straight bar or broom handle, which is placed squarely across your shoulders with the loop of the tied band placed under your feet.

Keep your body weight over the back portion of your foot rather than your toes; if needed, lift your arms out in front of you to shoulder height to balance yourself.

Begin squatting down but stop before your thighs are parallel to the floor (at about a 70-degree bend), keeping your back flat and your abdominal muscles firm at all times.

Hold that position for a few seconds before pushing up from your legs until your body is upright in the starting position.

Do squats with your back against a smooth wall if needed to maintain your balance.

3
KNEE DIPS

Equipment: exercise mat (optional)
Main muscles worked: quads, hamstrings, gluts, calves

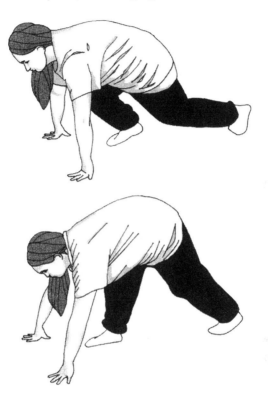

Directions:

Get into a sprinter's position facing forward as though you were at the starting line of a race, with one leg forward and one behind and your hands on the floor in front of you.

Bend both legs as much as is comfortable, bringing your knees as close to the floor as possible without touching.

Push your body upward until your legs are almost straight without locking your knees.

Switch the position of your legs and repeat.

4

KNEE LIFT

Equipment: resistance band, exercise mat (optional)
Main muscles worked: quads, hip flexors, abdominals

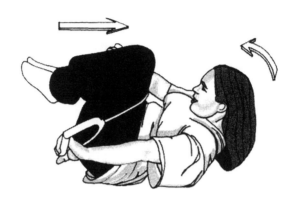

Directions:

Lie on your back with your knees bent.

Bend at your hip until your bent knees are positioned straight up over your hips at about a 90-degree angle.

Tighten your abdominal muscles to hold your lower back flat against the floor.

Lift your head slightly off the floor and position the resistance band across the front of your thighs, just above the knees.

Holding the band in your hands, stretch it by pulling your hands out more to the sides.

Pull your knees in toward your chest against the band to increase the resistance against your lower abs and the front of your thighs.

Slowly return to the starting position.

If holding your head slightly off the floor during this exercise is too hard, relax your neck muscles and rest your head on the floor.

5

SEATED LEG EXTENSIONS

Equipment: chair, resistance band or ankle weights (optional)
Main muscles worked: quads

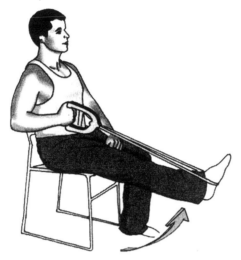

Directions:

Sit on the chair with your back straight and your feet and knees shoulder-width apart.

If using additional resistance, place the band around the bottom of your right foot with your knee bent (or put the ankle weight on), and then put your foot back on the floor.

Holding both ends of the band in your right hand, or, without any extra resistance, slowly straighten your right knee and lift your foot (without moving at your hip) until your leg is straight out in front of you (at a 90-degree angle to your torso).

Slowly bend your right knee and return to the starting position.

Repeat with the left leg.

6
STANDING LEG CURLS

Equipment: wall or stable chair back, resistance band (optional)
Main muscles worked: hamstrings

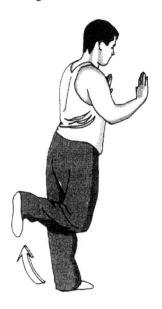

Directions:

Stand next to a wall or other support with your hands on it more than shoulder-width apart, and then bend your right knee.

Keeping your knees close together, smoothly lift your right heel up toward your bottom.

Hold your heel as close to your bottom as you can lift it for several seconds before returning your foot slowly to the floor.

To increase the intensity of the curl, place a resistance band around your right ankle with your knee bent, and hold both ends of it with your right hand during the movement.

Repeat with the left leg.

7

STANDING SIDE LEG RAISES

Equipment: wall or stable chair back, resistance band (optional)
Main muscles worked: gluts, outer thigh

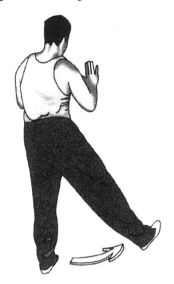

Directions:

Stand behind a chair and hold onto the back or place your hands shoulder-width apart on the wall.

Lift your right leg straight out to the side until your foot is about 6 to 12 inches off the floor, and hold for several seconds.

Keep your torso erect throughout the movement, and slightly bend the leg that is supporting your weight.

Return your leg to the starting position.

For added resistance, tie your resistance band into a circle and place it around both of your ankles before lifting one leg at a time out as far as you can against the band.

Repeat with your left leg.

8

CALF RAISES

Equipment: stair or ledge, dumbbells (optional)
Main muscles worked: calves

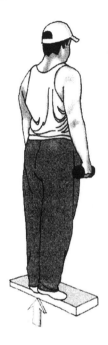

Directions:

Stand erect with the balls of your feet on a stable elevated surface (stair or ledge).

If using dumbbells, hold a dumbbell in one or both hands.

Keeping your body straight, balance on the ball of your foot and lift your heels as high as possible for several seconds.

Slowly lower your heels down as far as possible (even past being level with the stair or ledge, if possible).

Alternately, work one calf at a time, with or without holding a dumbbell.

More At-Home Versions for Lower-Body Exercises

HAVE FUN with these versions, or try using other household objects for variety.

Beach towel one-leg press (lower-body exercise 1): Try using a beach towel or sheet in place of the resistance band for the one-leg presses.

Olive oil squats (lower-body exercise 2): Do your squats while holding a bottle of olive oil (or other filled bottle or jar) in each hand.

Grandchild knee dips (lower-body exercise 3): Once you are in the sprinter's position, have a reasonably small child climb onto your back for the remainder of the exercise to add weight.

Blanket knee lifts (lower-body exercise 4): Do your knee lift using a rolled-up blanket or sheet instead of a resistance band.

Dictionary leg extensions (lower-body exercise 5): Find a dictionary or other heavy hardcover book, open it to the middle, and balance it over the bottom of your shin and across your ankle to add weight to your extensions.

Encyclopedia leg curls (lower-body exercise 6): Try using a heavy book to enhance your leg curl work by balancing it (open to the middle) across the bottom of your calf and over your heel while you do your repetitions.

Water-bottle side leg raises (lower-body exercise 7): Use a water bottle in a holder with Velcro straps, and secure the bottle (with varying amounts of water in it) to the outside of your ankle during side leg raises.

Soup-can calf raises (lower-body exercise 8): Hold a soup can in each hand while doing calf raises (or try larger cans, jars, or bottles for more weight).

Building a strong "core" and improving your balance

VIRTUALLY EVERYONE, you and I included, will develop some degree of lower back pain at some point in our lifetime. Walking around with an excessively big belly causes unusual stress on your lower back region and can contribute to discomfort. Moreover, if you already have a lower-back injury, inactivity is the best way to promote atrophy of the muscles in that area and increase the likelihood of having prolonged disability and recurrent injuries. The ability to balance and remain upright, essential for the prevention of falls and further injury, also diminishes as you allow your core and other muscles to weaken.

Building your core muscles. To prevent all types of injuries, promote better posture, and enhance balance, it's vitally important to include exercises that build and enhance a strong body "core." Building this core involves strengthening and stretching your lower back and abdominal regions equally, which can be done with various exercises. Keep in mind that your lower back has a relatively small amount of muscle compared to your front abdominal region, making it easier to work on your abs. Don't make the mistake of underemphasizing the strengthening of the lower-back muscles you do have, though, just because working your abs is easier.

Enhancing your lower-body strength is also an important part of preventing injury. When doing any upright exercises, lower your center of gravity for balance and injury prevention by bending at your hips and/or knees to absorb much of the muscular work in your lower body and to assist in keeping your back straight. Even when you pick up a light object off the floor, you'll want to practice such techniques to prevent straining your relatively weak lower back. The proper way to pick up any object from the floor is to bend your knees and flex your hips while keeping your lower back straight as you lower yourself down with your legs to reach the item. For a proper lifting technique, practice exercise 6 (suitcase lift) in the following section.

Using resistance training machines that isolate your lower-back region can further reduce your risk of lower-back injuries. If you have access to a back extension machine, by all means use it regularly. Practicing good posture at all times (sitting up straight, bending your knees whenever possible to reduce lower-back stress, and using chairs that provide lower-back support) can also help prevent lower-back pain and injury.

A word of caution about some of the following exercises: when doing abdominal crunches, you may feel pain in your neck because your abdominal muscles are weak and your neck muscles are helping to lift your upper torso. One way to relieve the stress on your neck is to take a towel, roll it up, and place it behind your head, and then hold both ends tightly so that the towel supports your neck. Keep the towel taut as you do any sort of curling-up abdominal work.

Abdominal/Lower-Back Exercises

1
CRUNCHES

Equipment: exercise mat (optional)
Main muscles worked: abdominals

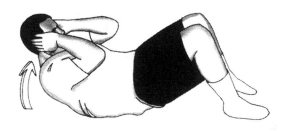

Directions:

Lie down on your back with your knees bent.

Place your hands on your head right behind your ears.

While breathing out, contract your abdominal muscles to lift your head, neck, and shoulders off the floor and curl forward no more than 45 degrees.

Hold for a moment before returning to the starting position, then repeat.

2
WAIST WORKER

Equipment: exercise mat (optional)
Main muscles worked: abdominals (obliques)

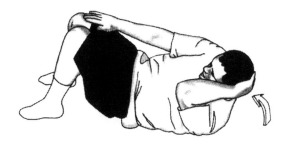

Directions:

Lie on your back on the mat with your legs bent, your feet flat on the floor, and your left hand behind your head.

Stretch your right hand across your body toward your opposite (left) knee and circle your hand three times around your knee in a counterclockwise direction; your right shoulder blade will lift off the mat.

Repeat the circular movement around the right knee using your left arm, but in a clockwise motion.

Keep your head in a neutral position and relax your neck to ensure that the contraction is in your abdomen area only.

3

CHAIR SIT-UPS

Equipment: chair or bench, resistance band (optional)
Main muscles worked: lower back

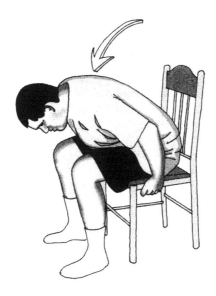

Directions:

Sit up straight in a chair with your feet on the floor, hands to your sides for support.

Bend forward, keeping your lower back as straight as possible, moving your chest down toward your thighs.

Slowly straighten back up, using your lower back muscles to raise your torso.

For added resistance, put a resistance band under both feet before you start and hold one end in each hand during the movement.

4

LOWER BACK STRENGTHENER

Equipment: exercise mat (optional)
Main muscles worked: lower back, gluts

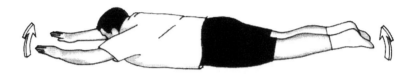

Directions:

Lie on your stomach with your arms straight over your head, your chin
resting on the floor between your arms.

Keeping your arms and legs straight, simultaneously lift your feet and
your hands as high off the floor as you can (aim for at least three
inches off the floor).

Hold that position (sort of a Superman flying position) for 10 seconds
if possible, and then relax your arms and legs back onto the floor.

If this exercise is too difficult to start, try lifting just your legs or arms
off the floor separately—or even just one limb at a time.

5

PELVIC TILT

Equipment: exercise mat (optional)
Main muscles worked: lower back, lower abdominals

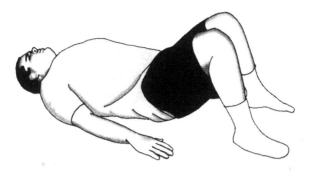

Directions:

Lie on your back on the floor with your knees bent, feet flat on the floor, and hands either by your sides or supporting your head.

Firmly tighten your bottom, forcing your lower back flat against the floor. Relax and repeat.

6

SUITCASE LIFT
(or, the proper way to lift items from the floor)

Equipment: dumbbells or household item, exercise mat (optional)
Main muscles worked: lower back, lower body (muscles involved in squats)

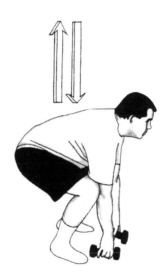

Directions:

After placing the dumbbells or household items slightly forward and between your feet on the floor, stand in an upright position with your back straight.

Keep your arms straight, with your hands in front of your abdomen.

With your back straight, bend only your knees and reach down to pick up the dumbbells.

Pick up the dumbbells or items in both hands, then push up with your legs and stand upright, keeping your back straight.

Balance enhancement. Maintaining your balance is important during almost all physical activities, and your ability to balance may diminish as you age. Research has shown, however, that loss of strength in your hips, knees, and ankles has a lot to do with your diminishing ability to balance, which means that it can be enhanced with specific exercises to strengthen those muscles. While core exercises can help with balance, other muscles are critical as well and should be worked with balance exercises. Specifically, the most important muscles for good balance are the ones that lift your legs to the side, the ones that lift your toes, and the ones that keep you moving forward. The primary "abductor" that lifts your legs to the side is a gluteal (buttocks) muscle, the gluteus medius; the main toe lifter is the tibialis anterior, on the front of your shins; and the primary muscle for maintaining forward movement is the gastrocnemius in your calves.

It's easy to lose your balance when you're standing or walking. Your head, trunk, and arms constitute two-thirds of your whole body weight, but with every step you take, that weight is carried and supported mainly by the hip muscles of your stationary leg. If these muscles are weak, they will allow you to tilt to the side, and if you slip when you're already tilted, you'll likely fall down. You can prevent this from happening, though. Side leg raises (lower-body exercise 7) are the best exercise to strengthen the abductor muscles of the upper thigh. Toe raises (listed as an additional balance exercise, below) can be done anytime, either sitting or standing, with one leg held out in front of you, to improve your toe-lifting ability. In addition, the calf raise (lower-body exercise 8) will strengthen the toe flexor muscles that keep you moving forward. Try to balance on your toes during that exercise for optimal balance improvement.

Additional Balance Exercises

THESE EXERCISES will help you improve your balance, so do them as often as you like. If you need to, hold on to or brace your hand against a table, chair, wall, or other sturdy object when you begin. As you progress, first use only one fingertip, and then try to do them without any support—as long as you have something sturdy nearby to hold on to should you become unsteady.

Toe raises: Standing with your hand on the back of a chair or against a wall, straighten one leg so that your foot is off the floor in front of you and flex your ankle to point your toes up at the ceiling. Hold this position for as long as you can; relax; and repeat several times before switching to the other leg.

Stork stands: Stand on one foot for a minute, and then switch to the other one. You can practice doing this exercise anytime you are standing.

Line walks: Take a step forward by positioning your heel in a straight line just in front of the toes of the opposite foot. As you take each additional step, the heel of your front foot and the toes of your back one should be barely or almost touching.

Sit/stand exercise: Practice standing up and sitting down without using your hands or arms for support or balance.

Flexibility moves to set you free

Flexibility exercises in their simplest form stretch and elongate muscles. Good flexibility is as important a part of fitness as stamina. Muscles must be strong, but they also have to be long (as opposed to contracted) to work optimally. In fact, stretching can do a lot more for your figure than aerobic exercise, because flexibilty work results in a supple, toned, and streamlined body. Moreover, the benefits of greater flexibility may go beyond the physical to include stress reduction and promotion of a greater sense of well-being. Exercise disciplines which incorporate stretching with breath control and meditation include yoga, tai chi, and Pilates.

In creating your flexibility workouts and completing them a minimum of two to three times a week, it's again important to include stretches for all of the major muscle groups in your body. You will regain some of your flexibility by stretching regularly, although your gains may be ultimately limited by your genetic makeup, diabetes control, arthritis, and other variables. Nonetheless, my own research found that all people with type 2 diabetes experience flexibility gains by doing just eight weeks of stretching of their major upper- and lower-body muscles thrice weekly in conjunction with a moderate resistance training program.

Flexibility Training Dos and Don'ts

Do:

▶ Use a full range of motion around joints when stretching

▶ Complete at least one stretch per major muscle group, optimally holding each stretch for 15 to 30 seconds

▶ Stretch all parts of your body two to three days per week

▶ Complete equal stretching exercises on both sides of your body or a joint

▶ Breathe deeply during all stretches to relax your muscles more

Don't:

▶ Bounce during stretches, as doing so can cause muscle tears and joint injuries

▶ Forget to stretch opposing muscle groups equally (e.g., quads and hamstrings)

▶ Stretch to the point of causing sharp pain or intense discomfort

▶ Continue with a stretch if you feel a sharp or immediate pain in any joint or muscle

▶ Hold your breath or strain while stretching

To get the maximum benefit, perform each stretch slowly. Doing the exercises correctly, with good form, is much more important than doing them quickly. To have any lasting effect on the muscle being stretched, you need to hold the stretch for at least 10 seconds to start. The more regularly you stretch, the better you become at judging how far to take your body. Aim to increase the duration of your stretches, so that you are eventually able to hold them for up to 30 seconds, the point at which muscles optimally start to lengthen. Also, be sure to stretch both sides of your body equally, as well as opposing muscles on both sides of a joint (such as biceps and triceps on the upper arm).

TIP
22

--- **NO MATTER YOUR WEIGHT** ---

MANY STRETCHING exercises can be done standing, sitting, and/or lying down, and the benefits are similar regardless of your body position. Pick the position or positions that are most comfortable for your body size and shape.

Upper-Body Stretches

1

NECK STRETCH

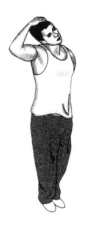

Stand with your feet apart and your knees slightly bent, or sit in a chair with your back straight and your feet on the floor. Relax your shoulders and gently bend your head toward your right shoulder. For an extra stretch, reach up with your right hand and apply a gentle pressure against the left side of your head in the direction of the stretch. Repeat on the left side. In addition, stretch your neck by tipping your head forward toward your chest and backward toward your spine.

2

SHOULDER/UPPER-BACK STRETCH

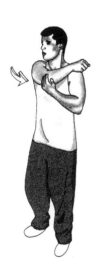

Stand with your feet a little apart, your knees slightly bent, and your stomach muscles slightly tensed. Relax your shoulders and pull your right arm horizontally across your chest by grabbing on to your elbow with your left hand. Repeat with your left arm. You can also do this exercise while seated in a chair.

3

CHEST/SHOULDER STRETCH

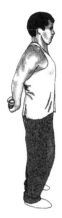

If standing, bend your knees slightly, tense your stomach muscles, and relax your shoulders; if seated, sit forward in your chair to make room for your arms to go behind you. Cross your hands behind your back and concentrate on bringing your shoulder blades toward each other as far as you can.

4

SHOULDER/BICEPS STRETCH

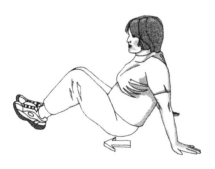

Sit on the floor with both legs extended out in front of you and your knees bent. Keeping your back straight, put your hands behind you with your palms flat on the floor and your fingers pointing away from your body. With your hands stationary, scoot your bottom forward until you feel the stretch in your shoulders, and then hold it.

5

UPPER BACK/TRICEPS STRETCH

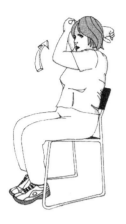

Sitting or standing, grab your right elbow with your left hand and push it straight up and back until the upper portion of your right arm is next to your right ear. Keep your spine and neck as straight as possible during this movement. Repeat with your left arm.

Lower-Body Stretches

1

QUAD (FRONT OF THIGH) STRETCH

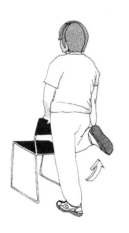

Holding on to a chair or the wall with your left hand, grab your right ankle with your right hand by bending at the knee, and bring your heel as close as you can toward your bottom (touching it, if possible). If that stretch is easy for you, then take it one step further by leaning forward slightly from that position and pulling your heel farther up and about six inches away from your bottom for maximum stretch. Repeat with the other leg. You can also do this stretch by lying on your side and stretching the top leg.

2

HAMSTRING (BACK OF THIGH) STRETCH

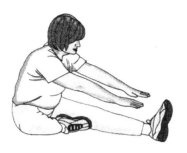

Sitting on the floor with your back straight, place your legs in a V. Next, bend your right knee and bring your foot in toward your groin area. Gently lean out over your left leg to stretch the back of your left thigh (don't worry if you aren't able to lean very far). Repeat with the other leg. Reminder: never bend your knee outward in the opposite direction (even though you may see other people doing so) to avoid injury to the knee joint.

3

GLUTS (BOTTOM) STRETCH

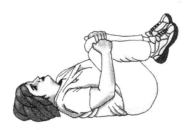

Lie on your back with both knees bent and your feet flat on the floor. Grab both of your knees with your hands and pull them up toward your chest as far as you can. Hold this position for several seconds before releasing. You can also do this stretch with one leg at a time.

4
CALF STRETCH

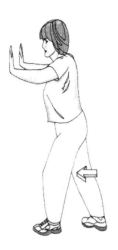

With straight arms, put your hands on a wall in front of you, and place your feet shoulder-width apart. Move your right foot about twelve inches more straight back while bending your left knee. Holding your back and your right knee straight, bend your elbows slightly and lean in a few inches toward the wall to stretch your right calf. Then, keeping your foot flat on the ground, slightly bend your right knee for an even greater stretch. Repeat this exercise with the other leg.

5
ABDOMINAL STRETCH

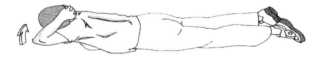

Lie down on your front with your arms over your head. Pull your arms in until you are propped up on your elbows. Gently arch your neck backward as far as is comfortable toward your bottom, keeping your hips on the floor. Hold the stretch for several seconds.

6
BACK/GLUTS STRETCH

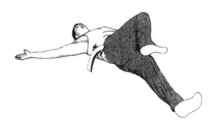

Lie down on your back with your arms straight out from your sides. Bend your right knee and then stretch it across your left leg while trying to keep your right hip on the ground. Repeat with the other leg.

7

COMPLETE BACK STRETCH (THE CAT STRETCH)

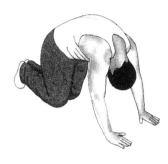

Kneel on all fours, keeping your knees in line with your hips, your hands in line with your shoulders, and everything in line with your spine, which should be flat. Breathe in as you slowly arch your back toward the ceiling with your abs tight, your pelvis tilted, and your gaze toward your navel. Breathe out as you reverse the action, drawing your chest toward the floor.

8

TOTAL BODY STRETCH

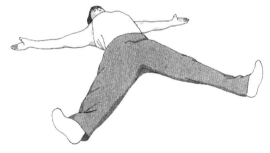

Lie on your back with your legs together and extend your arms straight up over your head on the floor. Tighten your abs and press your lower back firmly to the floor. Take a deep breath in and, as you breathe out, extend both your arms and legs as far away from your body and out to the sides as you can. Hold for several seconds before returning to the starting position.

Sample workouts to put it all together

No single routine or weekly workout plan will work for everyone, but a few examples follow. Use them as a starting point to help you individualize your own program of increased exercise, depending on your preferred physical activities. The exercise times recommended in the following plan can be decreased to 5 to 10 minutes at a time when you are just starting, and the days and types of activities can be varied accordingly. Some examples of variations are slow walking, brisk walking, cycling (outdoor or stationary), and swimming and other aquatic activities, just to name a few.

Remember, too, that at least one day of rest a week from your structured exercise plan—or at least a day when you do a different activity at a lower intensity—is optimal for muscle repair and will also result in fitness and strength gains, prevention of overuse injuries and overtraining, and sustainable motivation. For example, if you walk almost daily, your day of rest could include a completely different activity, like swimming or aqua aerobics. Feel free to actively engage in unstructured physical activity on your rest day.

Sample Structured Exercise Plan

Monday:
Moderate aerobic exercise (your choice) for 30 to 60 minutes, possibly done as two separate bouts of exercise (or two different activities)

Tuesday:
Resistance training, plus stretching and unstructured activities

Wednesday:
Moderate aerobic exercise for 30 to 45 minutes, with intermittent bouts of higher-intensity work interspersed at frequent intervals ("hard" day), plus some stretching

Thursday:
Easy aerobic exercise or unstructured activities for 45 to 60 minutes ("easy" day)

Friday:
Resistance training, plus stretching and unstructured activities

Saturday:
Mild to moderate aerobic exercise for 45 to 75 minutes (LSD day)

Sunday:
Rest day (unstructured activities only)

If you just can't find the time or the motivation to exercise at specific times and your preference is to simply add in more movement every day in an unstructured way, then the following plan is for you. Be creative and think of other activities that are more applicable to your lifestyle than the examples given, and make a conscious effort to incorporate them on a daily basis. Even if you choose to follow a structured exercise plan, continuing to add in more unstructured physical activity on a daily basis will only make you more fit and enable you to more effectively control your diabetes or prediabetes and your body weight. No matter how you do it, including more movement into each and every day is truly a necessity.

Sample Unstructured Exercise Plan

Weekdays (minimum added physical activity is 45 minutes a day):

Upon awakening—Completely tense whole body and relax 10 times (1 to 2 minutes)

Upon rising—Do warmup exercises 10 times each (e.g., toe touches, side bends, trunk twists, arm circles, neck rolls, knee lifts, calf stretches, jumping jacks (5 minutes)

On the way to work or other obligation—Park an extra distance away from your destination and walk, or arrive 5 minutes early and walk back and forth (5 minutes)

During work—Stand on your feet instead of sitting down whenever possible

After work—Upon arrival home, walk around the house five extra times before entering; if weather is inclement, walk the equivalent distance inside (5 minutes)

At home—Walk around for 5 minutes after every 15 to 20 minutes of a sedentary activity (and/or go up and down stairs) (5 to 15 minutes)

Before dinner—Set the dinner table, fill up drink glasses, or fix dinner (5 to 30 minutes)

After dinner—Clear the table and do dishes by hand (or load dishwasher) (5 to 10 minutes)

During evening leisure time—Walk in place or around during every TV commercial; if using a computer or reading, do the same for 5 minutes out of every 30 (10 to 30 minutes)

Before bedtime—Rise and lower on balls of feet while brushing your teeth; raise and lower your elbows while flossing (4 to 5 minutes)

Weekends (minimum added physical activity is 120 minutes daily):

Upon awakening—Completely tense whole body and relax 10 times (1 minute)

Upon rising—Do warmup exercises 10 times each (e.g., toe touches, side bends, trunk twists, arm circles, neck rolls, knee lifts, calf stretches, jumping jacks (5 minutes)

During morningtime—Walk around or in place during every TV commercial, if watching; if doing another sedentary activity, do the same for 5 minutes out of every half hour; also stand instead of sitting down whenever possible (20 to 30 minutes)

Before lunch—Take yourself and (possibly) the dog out for a walk (30 minutes)

After lunch—Go (window) shopping; park farther away on purpose, take the stairs, walk on escalators, etc. Alternately, go to the park, go for another walk, go for a bike ride, or do some gardening or yard work (40 to 60+ minutes)

Before dinner—Do household or other chores, such as vacuuming, sweeping, or cleaning up around the house (5 minutes)

After dinner—Turn on the stereo and dance or move during your favorite song (5 minutes)

During evening leisure time—Walk around or in place during every TV commercial; if using a computer or reading, do the same for 5 minutes out of every 30; also stand instead of sitting down whenever possible (10 to 20 minutes)

Before bedtime—Rise and lower on balls of feet while brushing your teeth; raise and lower your elbows while flossing (4 to 5 minutes)

Dealing with injuries or muscle soreness due to exercise

This discussion would not be complete without covering how to avoid injuring yourself and what to do about the inevitable muscle soreness you will experience after doing new or unaccustomed levels of exercise. You should expect some soreness or stiffness, but intense or lasting pain is not normal. If you do get injured (which you'll know due to the sharp, localized pain that you'll feel during or immediately after training), treat it with standard R.I.C.E. techniques—rest, ice, compression, and elevation—and then, as soon as the injury improves, ease slowly back into your exercise routine. Be sure to have the injury checked out by a physician if it doesn't start to get better within a week.

Types of injuries. Acute injuries may be caused by using improper exercise techniques or by carelessness (e.g., dropping a dumbbell on your foot), or they may be the result of excessive training that results in an overuse syndrome. The latter is the most nagging and persistently uncomfortable type of injury—kind of like having a pebble in your shoe that you can't get out. By definition, an overuse injury is caused by excessive use of a particular joint. As discussed previously, overuse injuries are more common in people with diabetes due to structural changes in their joints caused by elevations in BG levels over the long term. However, they are treated the same way regardless of how you get them.

Treatment of injuries. Overtraining is a common cause of shin pain, or "shin splints," which can be any number of conditions, including a stress fracture of the tibia (one of two shin bones) or inflammation occurring within a tissue or structure in that area. Using R.I.C.E. and possibly some anti-inflammatory medications such as ibuprofen (Advil or Nuprin) or naproxen sodium (found in Aleve), you should expect to see a decrease in your symptoms within a week of modifying your activities. If, however, you have tried these measures without experiencing any relief or have a single point of intense pain, you should see a physician (preferably a podiatrist who has expertise in foot, ankle, lower leg problems, and diabetes) who can further pinpoint the cause of your discomfort with an x-ray, bone scan, or MRI, if needed, and steer you to a more effective course of treatment that may include surgery, physical therapy, or rehabilitation of some type.

The important thing in dealing with activity-related injuries is to avoid going back to your normal activities until your symptoms have almost completely gone away. Cross-training is one way to deal with injuries without losing all of your conditioning while waiting for the injury to heal. For example, if you have lower leg pain, you can still work out your upper body doing other activities while allowing your legs to rest and recuperate. It is good during this time to alternate weight-bearing activities such as walking with non-weight-bearing ones, such as swimming and stationary cycling, so that you don't injure another part of your body.

Once you can resume your normal activities, work on strengthening the muscles around the affected area to prevent recurrence of the injury, particularly if it was the result of inflammation (as with tendonitis). For example, following a shoulder joint injury, you should focus on resistance work using all sections of the deltoid muscle, as well as biceps, triceps, pecs, and upper back and neck muscles, to strengthen muscles around the entire area.

General Tips for Safe and Effective Exercise

▶ Never bounce during stretches, as doing so can cause injuries.

▶ If you haven't exercised in a while, start out slowly and progress cautiously.

▶ Warm up with stretches and easy aerobic work before you begin to exercise more vigorously.

▶ Choose an exercise that suits your condition; for example, swimming might be better for those who find walking difficult.

▶ Find an exercise partner to help you stay motivated.

▶ Set goals to keep your interest up; for instance, if you walk for exercise, get a pedometer and set a goal of adding in 2,000 more steps each day.

▶ Reward yourself when you reach goals (but preferably not with food).

▶ Vary your exercise program occasionally or try out new activities; doing so also emphasizes different muscle groups and increases your overall fitness.

▶ Cross train to reduce the risk of injury by varying muscle usage.

▶ Wear appropriate shoes and socks, and check your feet after you exercise.

▶ When you start a new exercise, check your BG levels before, during (if more than an hour), and afterward.

▶ Don't forget to warm up and cool down for best results.

Muscle stiffness and soreness. Feeling stiff or tight after training is neither uncommon nor cause for alarm. Simply remember to stretch out all of your tight muscles and joints after workouts. If you are slightly sore the day after exercise, some gentle warmup and cool-down exercises can also help. However, if you are so sore a day or two afterward that your mobility is limited, then you are likely experiencing **delayed-onset muscle soreness (DOMS)**. Although unpleasant, DOMS is different from an acute injury and requires no special treatment.

DOMS is caused by damage you did to your muscles during training—such as lifting too much weight, running downhill, or overdoing a new activity—and it causes mild to severe muscle stiffness, pain, and cramping. The micro damage to the structure of your affected muscles becomes inflamed, and it may take two to three days to reach its maximum point of pain and a week or more to resolve completely. Mild activity, stretching, gentle massage, hydrotherapy (such as getting into a hot tub), and anti-inflammatory medications can all help alleviate the pain and discomfort you are feeling, but the best healer is simply time. The good news is that your body responds with "stress" proteins that it builds into the repaired muscles, making it very hard to reach that same level of soreness in the same muscles for six to eight weeks afterward, even if you overdo it with them again.

THE BOTTOM LINE ON STEP 3
Become Even More Fit

▶ Both warming up and cooling down are important parts of a planned workout session.

▶ Your overall fitness level can be enhanced and injuries can be prevented by varying the type and intensity of exercise that you do.

▶ Regularly intersperse intervals done at a harder intensity into your activities to improve your endurance.

▶ Including resistance training exercises in your routine two to three days a week will optimize your muscle-mass gain and insulin sensitivity.

▶ Stretching regularly is important for maintaining the flexibility of your joints and muscles.

▶ Taking a break from your structured exercise routine one day a week will help prevent overuse injuries, but include unstructured activities every day of the week for BG control.

▶ Body "core" exercises are important for preventing injuries and improving your balance.

▶ Some muscle stiffness and soreness following new or unaccustomed exercise is to be expected, but most injuries are preventable.

So, what are the keys to starting out? Plan big and start small. Try using the strategies discussed in step 3 to begin implementing small changes in your lifestyle that will bring more physical activity into your daily life, and then use the additional strategies given in this step to become as physically fit as you possibly can be.

DIABETES FITNESS PLAN STEP 3
in a Nutshell

YOUR PHYSICAL fitness and diabetes control will benefit most from a varied exercise program that includes aerobic exercise of differing intensities, resistance training, regular stretching, body "core" exercises, and a weekly day of rest.

Adopt an Optimal Eating Plan

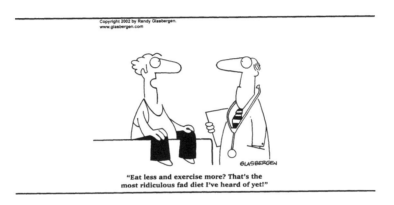

Copyright 2002 by Randy Glasbergen.
www.glasbergen.com

GLASBERGEN

"Eat less and exercise more? That's the
most ridiculous fad diet I've heard of yet!"

WHICH FAD DIET haven't you tried yet? Atkins? The South Beach Diet? The Hamptons Diet? Sugar Busters? The Cabbage Soup Diet? The Pineapple and Coconut Diet? (Okay, I admit I made that last one up.) Did you know that if you type in "diet" or "weight loss" into an online search engine such as Google, you get more than forty-two million hits for each one? Best-selling diets and diet books are a dime a dozen, and all they really do is lead to a lot of confusion about what constitutes good nutrition. Besides, if diets really worked, why would we need to keep trying so many different ones? Remember the earlier discussion on why "diet" is a four-letter word? If you remember nothing else, wrap your mind around this one point: diets don't work—at least not over the long haul—for almost anyone. If you truly want to become fit and to control your body weight and your diabetes, you are going to have to accept the fact that dieting is *not* an effective way to achieve or sustain your health goals—or to maintain a healthy emotional relationship to food in general.

Although healthier eating is undeniably important for your health, becoming more nutritionally fit will not necessarily coincide with any fad diet's mantra. What you do need to do is to adopt some healthier eating practices to go along with your more active lifestyle. So, before you swear allegiance to "low carb," "low fat," or any other unbalanced dietary plan, read the rest of this step to learn how better food choices are an integral part of achieving fitness with diabetes.

The importance of food choices in becoming fit

A research study hot off the presses strongly suggests that it is not carbohydrate per se that makes people gain weight, but rather the type of carbohydrate that they eat. Of 572 adults, those who ate more refined grains, starchy vegetables (such as white potatoes), white flour, and similar low-nutrition carbohydrates were significantly heavier than those who ate foods containing healthier carbohydrates, such as whole grains, non-starchy vegetables, and nuts and seeds. In short, body weights were higher in people who consumed more foods that are rapidly absorbed (i.e., those with a higher glycemic effect—more on this topic later) and cause spikes in BG (to more than 140 mg/dl).

I'm not the least bit surprised by the findings of that study; in fact, the results are exactly what I would have expected. Since I have researched only the effects of exercise and not of diet, how could I possibly have predicted the outcome in advance? It's easy, really: that study's findings reflect what we already know about the benefits of healthier carbohydrates and higher fiber intake as well as my personal experiences with controlling my BG while eating different types of carbohydrates. All carbohydrates should never be taboo, but we can certainly benefit from limiting our intake of more **refined carbohydrates**.

The food guide pyramid goes sideways

What may be most confusing about trying to figure out what you're supposed to eat is that even the supposed experts cannot agree on the best type of diet or meal plan. Although it was criticized for doing so, the federal government decided in 2005 to keep the pyramid shape of its original 1992 **Food Guide Pyramid**, which emphasized carbohydrate intake (represented by the base of the pyramid), while making only some cursory changes to encourage healthy eating and exercise. To wit, they flipped the pyramid on its side so that it is now divided top to bottom by six different-colored bands representing various food groups, with a set of steps beside it and a stick figure walking up them to emphasize exercise. Food proportions are represented by the different widths of the bands, with grains (orange) the largest, followed by dairy (blue), vegetables (green), fruits (red), meat and beans (purple), and fats (yellow). The actual portions you should eat on a daily basis to maintain your weight, however, depend on your age, sex, and amount of daily exercise.

Some health experts immediately criticized the new symbol, called "My Pyramid" (accessible at www.mypyramid.gov), for being more confusing than the old pyramid and for placing the primary responsibility for creating a slimmer, healthier America on consumers and not on food companies. They charged the government with catering to the food industry and special interest groups. The critics also claimed it would not help poorer Americans without easy access to a computer since you must access My Pyramid online to find out which of the twelve personalized pyramids is most applicable to you. My feeling is that, although it's not perfect, the government's improved pyramid does strive to emphasize healthier eating and more physical activity. It recommends that you make half of your grain intake whole grains to increase fiber; restrict your dairy intake to low- or nonfat varieties; add in more dark green and orange vegetables and legumes; eat a variety of fruit while limiting fruit juices; eat more fish, nuts, and seeds and lower the fat content of other protein sources; limit solid fat sources while making more of your fat selections from fish, nuts, and vegetable oils; and better balance your physical activity (30 minutes daily) and your food intake. Remarkably, this pyramid is the first guide that strongly addresses healthier types of fats and fiber intake.

What are you supposed to eat, really?

Only adding to the bewilderment of anyone with diabetes or prediabetes, both the American Diabetes Association and the American Dietetic Association still refrain from advocating any particular diet or food plan for weight loss and weight maintenance and choose not to formally recognize the importance of restricting certain foods, such as refined grains or **added sugars**, for optimal prevention or treatment of diabetes. As a person with diabetes myself, I strongly object to their lack of conviction about the glycemic effect of certain carbohydrates and foods. Although I'm not at all convinced that restricting the amount of carbohydrate in your diet is really that important if you're eating the right kinds of carbohydrates, I do know from personal and professional experience that what you eat does make a difference to your BG control. Nevertheless, just to increase your confusion, for every proponent of a "balanced" meal plan that follows the latest dietary recommendations of 45 to 65 percent of calories from carbohydrates (with the remaining 20 to 35 percent of calories from fats and 10 to 35 percent from protein), you'll find an equally fervent supporter of a lower-carbohydrate (40 percent of calories or less) plan.

For example, a recent study of obese people with diabetes who went on the Atkins (low-carbohydrate) diet reported that it caused rapid weight loss not because of increased water losses, changes in metabolism, or boredom with allowed foods, but because one consumes fewer calories by cutting carbohydrate intake down to 20 grams or less daily. The researchers concluded that carbohydrate intake drives excessive calorie intake, but that point, in my opinion, is debatable. There is no doubt, however, that the long-term healthiness of low-carbohydrate diets is dubious at best. Furthermore, a high protein intake may have particularly negative health consequences for you as excess protein can lead to the thinning of bones (which are already thinner if you have diabetes) and greater protein excretion by the kidneys (which may damage them long-term), not to mention a higher incidence of kidney stones and gout.

In contrast to that study, the same researchers reported in another research journal that people with type 2 diabetes lose similar amounts of weight on either of two more moderate diets: a "high-protein diet" (with 40 percent of calories coming from carbohydrates and 30 percent each from protein and fat), or a "high-carbohydrate diet" containing 55 percent carbohydrate, 15 percent protein, and 30 percent fat calories (which, incidentally, meets the current recommended intake of all three nutrients). Even though the high-carbohydrate diet contained 15 percent more carbohydrate calories than the high-protein one (which, incidentally, is not that big of a difference), it actually improved the participants' insulin sensitivity, fasting BG levels, and overall diabetes control more after eight weeks. Weight loss among the two diets was identical. From that study, you would *never* conclude that eating the recommended amount of carbohydrate is bad for diabetes control; on the contrary. Once again, it's the type of carbohydrate you eat that plays a significant role in its metabolic effects.

Joslin's guidelines can help lead the way

In the spring of 2005, the Joslin Diabetes Center in Boston, well respected for its role in the treatment of diabetes for over a century, finally took the lead and came out with its own version of diet and exercise guidelines for overweight people with either type 2 diabetes or pre-diabetes. The results of their scientific perusal of the most current research, Joslin's clinical guidelines (available at www.joslin.org/Files/Nutrition_ClinGuide.pdf), are intended to provide clear and easy-to-follow recommendations to improve insulin sensitivity and cardiovascular health while reducing body fat.

In brief, these guidelines recommend that less than 40 percent of daily calories come from carbohydrates (with a minimum of 130 grams of carbohydrate daily), 20 to 30 percent from protein (except in the presence of kidney problems), and 30 to 35 percent from fat (mostly mono- and **polyunsaturated fats**), along with a minimum of 20 to 35 grams of fiber (with a goal of 50 grams, if tolerated). They also advocate reducing daily caloric intake by 250 to 500 calories a day to allow most individuals to gradually lose no more than a pound every one to two weeks, but stress that minimum total daily calories should be 1,000 to 1,200 for women and 1,200 to 1,600 for men. Finally, they recommend a target of 60 to 90 minutes of moderate-intensity physical activity, including cardiovascular, stretching, and resistance activities, most days of the week, with a minimum of 150 to 175 minutes weekly.

As a whole, these guidelines are probably the most health-promoting ones that have ever been endorsed for prevention and control of type 2 diabetes. Although no foods are considered completely taboo in their plan, they do advocate that you consume fewer carbohydrates with higher glycemic effect, thus limiting your intake of refined carbohydrates or processed grains and starchy foods—especially pasta, white bread, low-fiber cereal, and white potatoes. Although they don't specifically say so, their endorsement of a 40 percent carbohydrate diet very likely stems from the fact that, as a whole, Americans are not likely to remove enough refined carbohydrates from their diet to effectively moderate the glycemic effect of eating more than 40 percent of their calories as carbohydrates.

The bottom line of Joslin's guidelines is that if you emphasize healthier sources, you will not need to cut all carbohydrates out of your diet (I certainly don't), and the same applies to fats and proteins, as long as you choose better types of fats and healthier sources of protein. Balanced meal plans, rather than extreme ones, are undeniably the best ones to follow—whether you have diabetes or not.

TIP
23

──────────── NO MATTER YOUR WEIGHT ────────────

AS THE debate about low- versus high-carbohydrate eating rages on and dietary fads come and go, the best approach in choosing a healthy meal plan for yourself is to realize that the actual composition of carbohydrate, fat, and protein in the foods that you eat is not nearly as important as the effect that individual foods have on your BG levels.

The glycemic index (GI) concept

Two important concepts will help you predict and control your BG response to your carbohydrate intake. The first of these is the **glycemic index** (GI). To their credit, the Joslin Center's guidelines are the first in the United States to actually mention the concept of GI in better meal planning. The **GI value** of a particular food is simply the effect it has on your BG levels. When you consume a carbohydrate, your body breaks it down through digestion and then absorbs it. The more rapidly it does so, the sooner the absorbed end-products of carbohydrates (mainly glucose) get into your bloodstream. GI values compare equal quantities of available carbohydrate in foods and are usually scaled from 0 to 100, with glucose being the most rapidly absorbed—its GI value is 100. If a food has a high GI value, then your BG will rise more rapidly after eating it; a lower number means that the food causes less of an immediate increase. While the actual range for each GI category may vary somewhat, "high-GI" foods are usually considered to be those with a GI value of 70 or more. These foods cause rapid rises in BG that are even harder to control if you have diabetes or insulin resistance.

Most of the foods in the high-GI category contain large amounts of highly refined flour or added sugars, including most ready-to-eat breakfast cereals, pretzels, sugary candy, and bread. White potatoes, though not a processed food, also fit into this list because they are digested so rapidly.

To deal with the influx of glucose from carbohydrates with higher GI values, your pancreas must be able to respond by releasing a large amount of insulin to take the resulting glucose out of your bloodstream and into cells around your body. Unfortunately, most people with diabetes lack the ability to respond to these glucose spikes with adequate amounts of insulin, as do many people with prediabetes and insulin resistance.

Other carbohydrate sources cause less of a spike in BG levels and are generally easier for your body to handle—depending on how much of them you eat. "Medium-GI" foods such as sweet potatoes, rice (white or brown), oatmeal, and white sugar have GI values in the range of 55 to 70. Any food with a GI value less than 55 is considered "low-GI"; examples are most whole fruits (since the GI value of fructose is not that high—even though it's a simple sugar), dairy products, legumes (beans), and pasta (white or whole-wheat). A more comprehensive list of GI values of common American foods taken from the International Table of Glycemic Index and Load Values (2002) can be found in Appendix C.

Other factors affecting GI

Your individual glycemic response to a particular food is affected by many factors, such as its fat and protein content, the type and amount of carbohydrate it contains, the amount of fiber and the nature of any starches in it, its preparation (raw or cooked), its ripeness, and even its acidity. In addition, the exact response to a particular food can vary considerably between individuals, just as metabolism does. While you may be able to easily understand why the higher fiber content of whole-grain bread makes it more slowly digested than a French baguette made of white flour, not all GI differences may be quite as obvious. For example, the glycemic response to diced potatoes is somewhat lower than to mashed potatoes, and thick linguine has a lower GI value than thinner spaghetti. Moreover, cooking in general—and particularly overcooking of foods—can raise their GI value, so al dente pasta is always better. Values for many ripe fruits (such as bananas), though, are actually lower than their greener, unripe precursors. Highly acidic foods, such as vinegar, can lower the GI value of another food when they are eaten in combination.

Critics of the GI concept like to point out that GI rankings reflect glycemic responses only over a two-hour time span after a particular food is eaten and that individual responses to any given food may vary widely.

Such debates over the GI have led some to conclude that low-GI diets are not necessarily effective for BG control or diabetes prevention because the GI value of a particular food may or may not reflect its entire glycemic effect. However, what's important to remember is that GI testing of foods is performed on people who are diabetes free. Moreover, an excessive intake of high-GI carbohydrate foods has been shown to increase insulin resistance even in people *without* diabetes. Because people with diabetes generally lack the ability to immediately release enough insulin in response to food intake (their "first phase" secretion), GI tables more than likely underestimate, rather than overestimate, the glycemic spikes caused by most carbohydrate-rich foods if you have diabetes.

How GI affects diabetes control

If you are already prediabetic, a high-GI food will have an even greater effect on your BG levels than on those of someone whose insulin works normally. When your insulin does not work properly, your BG will spike even higher in response to eating a high-GI food. Moreover, when you eat such foods can also have an effect. For example, your glucose levels will rise more following lunch if you ate a high-GI breakfast rather than a low-GI one—despite a greater release of insulin. Thus, the glycemic effect of eating a higher-GI carbohydrate first thing in the morning potentially lasts later into the day as well.

In overweight adults, insulin resistance can also be decreased by the consumption of a low-GI, whole-grain diet (rather than a refined-grain, "white" diet), regardless of your level of excess body fat. Moreover, type 2 diabetic men following a low-GI diet (consuming mostly foods with a GI value of under 40) are also able to improve their BG control, enhance their insulin action, and lower their levels of blood fats after only four weeks on such a meal plan. Such positive results overwhelmingly give credence to the argument that the GI is an appropriate guide to eating more nutritious foods whether you have diabetes, prediabetes, or insulin resistance.

The effects of fat on GI values

Although a higher fat content lowers the immediate effect of most foods on your BG (for example, the GI value of a baked potato is higher than that of potato chips), many types of fat are actually detrimental to your metabolism and can cause insulin resistance on their own. In particular, **saturated fats** (solid at room temperature), such as those found in abundance in red meat, butter, dairy fat, and tropical oils (palm and coconut), decrease insulin action and result in higher BG levels. Trans fats, which are created during manufacturing and are commonly found in margarines, crackers, baked goods, and other processed foods, have a similarly negative effect on insulin action; luckily for consumers, manufacturers are now required by law to list trans-fat content on food labels and, accordingly, many foods are now being made with fewer of these heart-unhealthy fats.

Combination foods with significant carbohydrate and fat content, such as pizza, have a lower GI value because the fat slows down the absorption of the carbohydrates, so that it takes longer than two hours for the pizza to be metabolized and fully exert its effects on your BG levels. While eating this fat load may initially slow down your carbohydrate absorption, its later glycemic effect should not be discounted. The saturated fat in pizza, for example, will make you more insulin resistant four to five hours later, when it finally hits your circulation and reduces your uptake of glucose. The heightened state of insulin resistance that results raises your BG level and worsens your glycemic response to high-GI foods the next time you eat.

Thus, despite its medium-GI value, pizza—with its high content of refined carbohydrates and saturated dairy fat—is best eaten only in very small quantities (no more than one to two slices), and you should eat plenty of salad or another low-GI, low-fat, high-fiber food along with it. Thankfully, healthy fats such as those found in fish, nuts, and olive oil don't appear to similarly increase levels of insulin resistance.

Can you really eat all the sugar you want to?

Despite research showing that people with diabetes are able to control their BG better when they limit their intake of all sources of refined (high-GI) carbohydrates, most health-care professionals have relaxed their stand on sugar consumption (particularly if you have type 1 diabetes or take insulin for every meal). This is because research has shown that some "simple" sugars (such as table sugar, a.k.a. **sucrose**, a **disaccharide** composed of two simpler sugars—a glucose molecule and a fructose one—both of which are **monosaccharides**) are actually metabolized more slowly and have a lower GI value than certain "complex" carbohydrates (including starches like white potatoes). They advise you to focus instead on counting and limiting the total grams of carbohydrates from any source that you eat, both at any given meal and over the course of a day.

While the GI value of white potatoes does exceed that of sucrose, I still think that this stance is giving people the wrong idea about the potential effect that certain carbohydrates can have on your BG control. Let me give you a personal example. For me, by far the worst thing about getting diabetes at the age of four was not the shots I had to get, but rather being forced to abandon my favorite cereal, sugary Froot Loops. Back in the "dark ages" when I got diabetes (1968), the health-care providers' mantra was, "You can't eat any sugar." Back then, people even thought that eating too much sugar was the cause of type 2 diabetes.

Nowadays, although in accordance with this more modern-day stance on sugar intake I would once again be allowed unrestricted access to my formerly beloved Froot Loops, you couldn't pay me enough to eat them (well, not unless I needed to treat a low BG level). Why? Well, in spite of not really liking the taste anymore, I choose not to eat that cereal because its high GI value would invariably cause me to chase my BG down with much higher doses of insulin than I ever take in the morning for an equivalent amount of carbohydrate from my habitual oatmeal-and-fresh-fruit breakfast. To me, Froot Loops cereal (and most other breakfast cereals, for that matter) is just not worth the inevitable spike in my BG and the extra insulin I'd have to take to try to control it. If you have type 2 diabetes, your body just won't be able to supply that extra insulin quickly enough. So, would I ever advise you to substitute a sugary food in place of a more slowly absorbed one with equivalent carbohydrates? Never. Such substitutions also ignore the satiety factor—the fact that you'll feel fuller and more satisfied after a high-fiber breakfast of oatmeal and fruit than you ever would after eating a sugary cereal. (I'd also advise you against eating instant oatmeal instead of the old-fashioned kind because the former contains a lot more sugar, which will sabotage your attempts to effectively control your BG levels.)

TIP

24

NO MATTER YOUR WEIGHT

CONTRARY TO popular belief, eating too much sugar is *not* a direct cause of diabetes; however, the effects of eating white sugar and other refined carbohydrates should not be discounted as harmless. Refined carbohydrates are a source of "empty calories" that contain few essential nutrients, lots of calories, and higher-GI carbohydrates certain to throw off your BG balance.

The glycemic load (GL) concept

The glycemic index works best when it is combined with the second concept for predicting the glycemic effect of your total carbohydrate intake, known as **glycemic load** (GL). GL takes into account both the GI value *and the quantity* of carbohydrates that you eat. A GL of 20 or more is "high," 11 to 19 is "medium," and 10 or less is "low." Foods that have a low GL almost always have a lower GI value, with some exceptions: watermelon has a high GI value (72), but the carbohydrate content per serving of this fruit is minimal, making its GL (4) low (but you do have to watch how big of a piece you eat, since a serving is just over a cup); popcorn also has a higher GI value (72), but it takes a lot to equal 50 grams, which have a GL of just 8.

A careful consideration of the GL of foods is crucial if you want to prevent type 2 diabetes. Several large-scale studies have now confirmed that eating a high-GL diet over the course of years substantially increases your risk for developing diabetes. In other words, overloading with "white" carbohydrates may actually contribute to its onset. Paying attention to your GL is even more important once you have diabetes, when you're attempting to achieve good control of your BG levels. New research has also shown that eating a low-GL, high-fiber diet raises circulating levels of adiponectin, an anti-inflammatory hormone released by fat cells. If you have diabetes, higher levels of adiponectin in your system will lead to improved insulin sensitivity, reduced inflammation, and better BG control.

Can pasta really have a low GL?

Unfortunately, you can't always believe what you read when it comes to the GL of processed foods. Despite what many food manufacturers would like you to believe with their "net carbs," "carb smart," and other misleading marketing claims that make foods like high-GL pasta appear to be almost carbohydrate free, the total amount of carbohydrate that you eat, particularly in a high-GL food, can't be discounted simply because it has a lower GI value. Slowly absorbed carbohydrates, such as those found in pasta, are still metabolized and contribute to your carbohydrate and calorie intakes for the day. I've seen packages of pasta that claim to have "only 5 net carbs" per serving, giving you the impression that you would only be eating 5 total grams of carbohydrate; in fact, the food label revealed that it actually contains 42 grams of carbohydrate per serving and only 2 grams of fiber.

Accordingly, despite the fact that most pasta has a lower GI value, if you eat more than half a cup of it (equal to one serving, which is a lot less than anyone usually eats at a time), the large carbohydrate load will still have a pronounced glycemic effect, and your BG may rise excessively. Read food labels carefully, though, as some companies have decreased the carbohydrate content of their pastas by adding in extra fiber—which you can determine by looking up the fiber content on the label. The grams of fiber are not absorbed and can be subtracted from the total carbohydrates listed for the product to determine its actual carbohydrate load (which will be affecting your insulin needs and BG levels).

TIP
25

--------- **NO MATTER YOUR WEIGHT** ---------

MODIFYING YOUR eating habits away from high-glycemic-load and higher-GI foods can help you reduce or reverse the symptoms of diabetes or prediabetes without weight loss and, as an added bonus, prevent you from gaining any more weight.

The combined importance of GI and GL

Since everyone with diabetes has trouble producing enough insulin to cover the BG spikes resulting from high-GI and high-GL meals and snacks, the best way to effectively manage your diabetes is to control both the type and amount of carbohydrates that you consume. This is the technique that I always employ. In fact, in my experience, to have effective control over your BG levels, you absolutely have to avoid overloading with carbohydrates, particularly ones with higher GI values.

Along the same lines, you get hungry again more quickly after high-GL meals than after low-GI and low-GL ones. This hunger may be the result of a drop in BG levels due to the greater insulin release that typically follows a large glycemic load or a sustained rise in BG if inadequate amounts of insulin are released by your pancreas in response to a meal like a big bowlful of mashed potatoes. When carbohydrates are absorbed more slowly, however, your BG will stay more constant, usually leaving you feeling satiated longer. For most people, a low GI/GL diet plan results in weight loss as well.

You can improve your BG control by either decreasing your body's need for insulin or improving your sensitivity to it. Elevated BG levels, however, create a greater demand for insulin, which in turn constantly overworks your pancreas. Although beta-cell insulin production declines as you age regardless of your ethnicity, it is not yet clear what causes the loss of beta-cell function over time. Is it primarily due to the exhaustion of these cells caused by a constant state of overwork when insulin resistance is high (and higher-GI foods are eaten)? Does their function deteriorate due to the presence of toxic levels of glucose that directly damage them? Or, is it a combination of both of these processes? Whatever the cause, though, if you're sedentary, overweight, prediabetic, and/or diagnosed with type 2 diabetes, a high-GI/GL diet will most likely exacerbate your insulin resistance and your body's ability to supply enough insulin.

When selecting the best foods to eat, take into account the glycemic effect, the total carbohydrate content, and the nutrient density of your meals and snacks. It's best to limit your intake of foods with both a high or medium GI value and a high GL (as listed in Appendix C). Any carbohydrate-rich meal (i.e., one with an overall high GL) will require the release of more insulin, but at least if the GI value is lower—as is generally the case with higher-fiber foods—the immediate rise in BG will be lessened, and you will likely feel satisfied longer.

Some researchers have also shown that diets with high GI values are associated with an increased risk of breast cancer among post-menopausal women who have used hormone replacement therapy and who are not overweight. The association appears to be even stronger among those women who do not engage in vigorous physical activity. In men, high GL and sucrose intake are related to an elevated colorectal cancer risk. So, after hearing all this, are you positive that you still want to eat a high-GI/GL diet?

TIP
26

─────────── **NO MATTER YOUR WEIGHT** ───────────

IF YOU have recently eaten foods with a high GL or high GI values, your body may have a harder time handling any additional, similar carbohydrates at your next meal or snack—unless you exercise first and use up a significant amount of your stored muscle glycogen. Glycogen-depleted muscles give the next carbohydrate load somewhere to go to get out of your circulation and be stored for later use.

Adding more fiber to your diet

No matter what your perception of fiber is, believe me when I say that it is far more than just something you need to eat to keep "regular." Actually, fiber is a collective term for the indigestible **polysaccharides** in our diets, both the natural ones in foods and others that come from "functional" sources extracted or isolated from foods or manufactured synthetically (such as Metamucil). As for its solubility in water, fiber is either soluble or insoluble. Soluble fiber, found in oatmeal, legumes, seeds, fruits (apples, bananas, citrus fruits), and vegetables, dissolves in water and is partially metabolized in the large intestine by "friendly" bacteria that normally reside there. This type of fiber may play a large role in removing cholesterol from the body. The insoluble form is found in vegetables (carrots, celery, and the skins of corn kernels), parts of fruit (apple peels, core, and seeds), brown rice, and whole grains (such as the outer membranes of wheat kernels). This fiber, acting as roughage, passes through your digestive system without being fully digested, primarily serving to increase fecal bulk and ensure regular elimination of bodily waste products. Since either type of fiber pulls some water out of your body, it is best to add an extra glass or two of water to go along with consumption of more fiber.

Despite the well-known fact that a high-fiber diet may help reduce your chances of developing heart disease, diabetes, obesity, strokes, colorectal and other types of cancer, diverticulosis, and hemorrhoids, most Americans still don't eat enough fiber. If you are at high risk of developing type 2 diabetes, a diet high in fiber can enhance your insulin sensitivity and help lower your risk. A portion-controlled, low-GI diet containing Mexican-style foods (pinto beans, whole-meal wheat bread, and low-GI fruits) can also improve glucose levels in obese people with type 2 diabetes due to its low GI value and high fiber content.

Fiber is also helpful because it generally slows down the rate at which food empties from your stomach, thus limiting rapid BG peaks. It also increases satiety, meaning that you feel full longer, which may help prevent excessive eating and weight gain. Foods that are higher in fiber are also, on the whole, lower in added sugars, fat, and calories. As discussed, the best strategy to control your diabetes is not to eliminate carbohydrates per se, but rather to eat higher-fiber carbohydrates— which means most of the foods with a lower GI value and lower GL. If you eat a low-fiber food like a candy bar, you will likely still feel hungry afterward despite an excessive intake of calories, and your BG will go up too much. If, on the other hand, you eat a high-fiber apple along with a small handful of nuts or a chunk of low-fat cheese, it will take you longer to eat, and in the end you will feel more satisfied despite having eaten fewer calories.

How much fiber do you need?

The generally recommended fiber intake for adults is 25 to 40 grams per day, depending on caloric intake (12.5 grams per 1,000 calories consumed), but Joslin's new nutritional guidelines recommend eating at least 50 grams of fiber a day, which is extremely optimistic given that most people don't even meet the currently recommended levels. Instead of getting caught up in trying to eat a certain amount of fiber daily, make it easier on yourself by simply making a steadfast commitment to eat more whole grains, fruits, vegetables, and legumes; your fiber intake will greatly increase (maybe even up to 50 grams a day). To find out the fiber content of any food, either read its nutrition label (if it comes in a box or package), or, for produce or natural foods, look up fiber information on a variety of nutrition-related Web sites via the Tufts Nutrition Navigator (http://navigator.tufts.edu). Although the low-carb craze has resulted in many new products with added fiber (such as pasta and tortilla shells), remember that in general, the more refined a product is, the less fiber it is likely to contain.

The Best Sources of Dietary Fiber

ALTHOUGH A product or a food item can only be labeled "high fiber" when it contains more than 5 grams of fiber per serving, many foods (all from plant sources) are good, healthy sources of dietary fiber:

▶ All dry peas and beans (legumes), including navy beans, garbanzo beans (chickpeas), lentils, black beans, kidney beans, soybeans, lima beans, and pinto beans.

▶ Vegetables, particularly green beans, snap beans, pole beans, beet greens, kale, collards, Swiss chard, turnip greens, spinach, peas, broccoli, Brussels sprouts, tomato paste, carrots, and corn.

▶ Dried fruits, such as apricots, figs, and dates (but all of these have a high carbohydrate content).

▶ Whole fruits (with skins, but not peels), including raspberries, blackberries, strawberries, blueberries, cherries, plums, pears, oranges, apples, bananas, kiwi fruit, and guava.

▶ Whole-grain foods such as rye, oats, buckwheat, brown rice, whole-wheat breads and pasta, oat and wheat bran, high-bran-content cereals (e.g., All-Bran), soy flour, and popcorn.

▶ Nuts and seeds, such as cashews, peanuts, almonds, Brazil nuts, walnuts, pecans, pistachios, and sunflower seeds (but all of these are also high in calories).

Foods—better consumed as nature intended

Nutrients in foods work best the way they are created in nature—that is, the way that they grew, or in combination with other vital ones that grew alongside them. Often it's not just the nutrients themselves that are vital, but also the synergy of their various activities in your body. Unfortunately, while foods are going through processing (as when whole wheat is processed into white flour, bleached or unbleached), numerous nutrients are stripped out, and only a select few are added back in by the manufacturers. The result is that processed foods are far less nutritious than foods eaten in a more natural state.

Go heavy on the phytonutrients

Fruits and vegetables are particularly rich in compounds called phytochemicals, which I prefer to call **phytonutrients**—naturally occurring substances found in plants that have disease-fighting and health-promoting powers. While phytonutrients such as capsaicin, lycopene, lutein, quercetin, saponins, and terpenes can't be bought in supplement form, consuming these nutrients in their natural form may provide an extra health benefit from the additive and synergistic combinations of these bioactive substances in whole foods that you would be unlikely to get from a supplement—if any were available. If you hate vegetables or avoid fruits in favor of sweeter desserts, keep in mind that a single serving is only a half cup of a cooked vegetable, a cup of melon or berries, or a medium-sized piece of fruit.

Certain foods containing phytonutrients may even one day cure diabetes. It was recently discovered that sweet and tart cherries increase insulin production in beta cells by 50 percent (but so far, this effect has only been proven in rodents). These cherries are apparently loaded with anthocyanins, which contribute to the fruit's bright red color. This phytonutrient can also be found in other bright red, blue, and purple produce such as red grapes, strawberries, and blueberries, as well as in wine, cider, and tea. So far, though, the biggest insulin-enhancing effects appear to come from the type of anthocyanins found in these particular cherries.

Color your food

For the first time ever, the USDA's 2005 food guide pyramid addresses eating produce of varying colors on a daily basis—which is quite an improvement, in my opinion. Americans have gotten into the bad habit of eating colorless foods, including white bread, white rice, white potatoes, white sugar, and white (iceberg) lettuce. A recent book, *The Color Code: A Revolutionary Eating Plan for Optimal Health*, discusses research on the health benefits of phytonutrients and recommends that you choose foods from a minimum of four color groups daily: red, orange-yellow, green, and blue-purple. The phytonutrients available in each color group vary with the pigment. For example, red foods such as tomatoes and tomato products contain lycopene, which may prevent prostate cancer in men; the carotenoids in yellow-orange foods may reduce your risk of heart disease; green foods such as broccoli contain sulforaphane, a cancer fighter; and blueberries, in the last color group, contain nearly one hundred different known phytonutrients, making them the number-one-ranked food in terms of **antioxidants** and disease-fighting power.

Generally speaking, the darker the food, the more phytonutrients it contains. Legumes illustrate this concept well: black beans are highest in antioxidants (flavonoids), followed by the red, brown, yellow, and white varieties, in decreasing amounts. The majority of these compounds are found in the darker-colored seed coats of the legumes; the outer coatings contain the antioxidants that plants use to protect themselves from oxidative damage by the sun's ultraviolet rays, and plants with more of these compounds are better protected.

The antioxidant punch of certain fruits and vegetables

Antioxidants are very popular supplements because of their purported ability to slow aging, which is believed to result largely from cumulative oxidative damage in the body. Since the majority of diabetic complications appear also to be related to unchecked **oxidative stress** in various tissues and organs, eating foods containing more antioxidant power may somewhat mitigate the negative impact of elevated BG. In addition to blueberries, go out of your way to include other particularly potent fruits with high antioxidant and disease-fighting power in your diet, including strawberries, raspberries, oranges, mangoes, grapefruit (particularly pink), kiwi, avocados, concord grapes, cherries, and dried plums.

The list of vegetables to embrace in your diet includes tomatoes and broccoli, as well as red bell peppers, sweet potatoes (number-one vegetable for overall content of vitamins A and C, folate, iron, copper, calcium, and fiber), carrots (number two), winter squash, kale, spinach, purple cabbage, and eggplant. As for other foods, dark chocolate and cocoa, red wine, green and black tea, and coffee also contain large amounts of antioxidants, but moderate your consumption of semisweet dark chocolate and wine to avoid taking in too many calories.

More general tips for healthier eating

Good nutrition is a balancing act requiring that eating foods with a higher GL be combined with limiting the total amount that you consume and with taking in more foods with a lower glycemic punch. You don't need to completely avoid all sugary or high-GI snacks—just learn to limit your consumption of them. One good tip is that if you don't buy certain foods, you won't be as likely to eat them. Also, limit the varieties of snack foods you buy, such as cookies or chips, because you will tend to eat more when a larger selection is available. If your only snack choice is one less-healthy snack food, you may tire of it and choose other, healthier options for variety. Instead of filling up on nutrient-poor, high-calorie foods, balance consumption of such items with an expanded intake of healthier snacks and meals with a higher satiety potential. For more help in making better selections, consult the food-buying guide in Appendix D.

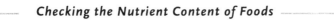

Checking the Nutrient Content of Foods

ONE WAY to eat healthier is to select foods that are higher in nutrient content for a given number of calories—meaning that they are "nutrient dense." You can easily check the nutrient content of any food for free by logging onto the USDA's Web site at http://www.nal.usda.gov/fnic/foodcomp and clicking on "Search the Nutrient Database." Their list of foods encompasses more than six thousand items, and each is analyzed for nearly 120 separate nutrients. By choosing the "Nutrient Lists" option, you can also search for single nutrients within foods, making it easier to identify foods high in desirable nutrients like calcium, iron, and fiber, as well as less desired elements like calories and saturated fat. It also allows you to check for the content of a limited number of phytonutrients, including **beta-carotene**, lutein, and lycopene.

Reducing refined and added sugar intake

One of the easiest ways to start improving the glycemic effect of your diet is to reduce or eliminate your intake of all regular soft drinks, juice, fruit-juice drinks, and other sugar-sweetened drinks such as iced tea or lemonade. It's infinitely better to substitute water, diet (newly renamed "zero") soft drinks (especially the non-caffeinated, non-cola varieties), other artificially sweetened beverages such as Crystal Light or Propel water, or small amounts of skim milk in their place. Why is it so important to cut back on sugary caloric drinks? By not drinking calorie-filled sodas, you're likely to consume 10 percent fewer calories than soda consumers on a daily basis. The negative effect of such drinks on diabetes control is an even more important issue, and your BG will suffer if you drink sugar-filled sodas or juices.

Cutting back on refined sugar in other foods involves being a more informed and careful consumer. You will need to identify sources of added sugars by reading food labels and checking all food ingredients carefully. By law, manufacturers must list ingredients in order of descending weight. In many products, that means sugar would come first, so companies have found many creative ways to disguise added sugars. Instead of using one source of added sugar, companies commonly add four or five different sweeteners so that each one will appear lower on the list of ingredients. So watch out for all the added sugar equivalents: sucrose, **dextrose**, high-fructose corn syrup, corn syrup, glucose, fructose, maltose, levulose, honey, brown sugar, and molasses.

Unfortunately, choosing "sugar-free" and "fat-free" varieties of foods is not necessarily better, either. Such products, especially "sugar-free" cakes, cookies, candy, and the like, are rarely sugarless (as you will discover when you scan the labels for all of the above-listed possible sugar equivalents), and most are far from being calorie free or even from having reduced calories. Such products are typically high in fat and not beneficial to anyone with diabetes. Along the same lines, "fat-free" products are usually higher in sugar. Just keep in mind that any time food manufacturers remove flavor enhancers such as fat or sugar, they have to replace them with something else; if fat is taken out, sugar is usually added in and vice versa.

Sugar alcohols are not necessarily better

Sugar alcohols are often promoted as being sugar alternatives, but products containing them are never "free" foods. Sorbitol and mannitol (and others that end in *ol*) are either absorbed more slowly or poorly absorbed to some extent (thus reducing their GI value), but they still contain almost the same amount of carbohydrate or GL. Sorbitol is often used as a sugar substitute in candy products such as "sugarless" gummy snacks, and except for taking longer to metabolize, the carbohydrate effects are similar to those of white sugar and with equivalent calories. (Incidentally, the malabsorbed part of most sugar alcohols has a laxative effect, so if you eat as much as 10 grams of sorbitol or mannitol at one sitting, make sure a bathroom is nearby.)

Similarly, lactilol, an altered form of milk sugar found in products such as Hershey's "sugar-free" dark chocolate candy bars, is neither truly sugarless nor calorie free. Its calorie content is equal to that of their regular chocolate bars, and a similar number of carbohydrates will eventually be absorbed, albeit more slowly. A slower rate of absorption may help control your diabetes better, but be careful not to overeat such "sugar-free" foods just because you mistakenly believe that they don't contain as many grams of carbohydrate or calories.

Try out some artificial sweeteners instead

On the other hand, when **artificial sweeteners** are used in diet soft drinks, flavored waters, ice cream, and many other products, the calorie content from the replaced added sugars may be substantially reduced or completely eliminated. These low-calorie sweeteners truly are "free" foods because they make food taste sweet without adding calories or affecting BG levels, and in meal planning, they do not count as a carbohydrate, fat, or any other exchange.

A number of artificial sweeteners have been approved for use by the FDA and likewise endorsed by the ADA. They currently include saccharin, aspartame, acesulfame potassium, sucralose, neotame, and tagatose, although new sugar substitutes are being tested and approved all the time. The most popular one currently on the market, a relative newcomer named sucralose (marketed as Splenda), has already largely replaced aspartame (NutraSweet) in many products. Some people are sensitive to NutraSweet and have negative reactions such as headache or stomach upset when they consume it. If that is the case for you, try Splenda or another sugar substitute instead.

TIP

27

───── **NO MATTER YOUR WEIGHT** ─────

ANY LOW-CALORIE sweetener may help you reduce your calorie intake and stick to a healthier meal plan, particularly if you are overweight or have diabetes. In addition, these sweeteners are particularly useful for reducing your intake of high-GI carbohydrates when used in place of sugar to sweeten coffee, tea, cereal, or fruit.

Choosing healthier fats is vital

Diabetes is actually a metabolic disorder related not only to BG abnormalities, but also to deleterious changes in blood fats. Elevations in blood levels of triglycerides (which mainly come from dietary fat) and cholesterol, particularly the less healthy LDL cholesterol that contribute to arterial plaque formation, are main players in the inflammatory process leading to the development of cardiovascular disease so common in people with diabetes.

Low-fat diets are not necessarily the answer, though. Such diets can actually cause an increased production of LDL cholesterol, especially when fat calories are replaced with highly refined carbohydrates. When people known to have high cholesterol go on one of two diets that are equally moderate in fat (30 percent of calories) and saturated fat (10 percent), their cholesterol levels go down far more when they eat more vegetables and fruits (13.5 daily servings versus only 5), beans and nuts (4 servings), and whole grains (3.5 servings), while consuming fewer prepared foods (such as lower-fat versions of snack foods and cheese). These findings demonstrate once again that not all forms of fat are metabolized equally or need be avoided.

Which fats are the better ones?

Recently, researchers showed that when a high-fat breakfast is eaten, if it contains mainly a "good" fat (for example, monounsaturated fat from olive oil) rather than a "bad" one (for example, saturated fat from cream or butter), then your body uses the consumed fat at a higher rate, glucose and insulin levels stay lower, and more energy is expended during its digestion. Diets rich in monounsaturated fats, which are the primary type of fat found in olive oil, canola oil, and nuts, are actually heart-healthy and do not necessarily promote weight gain or insulin resistance. In fact, if you're on a diet and eat a handful of almonds daily, you'll likely lose more weight than someone on another diet eating the same reduced number of calories but no almonds. Diets high in monounsaturated fats may also improve your insulin action.

There are two essential types of fat, but your intake of them will vary widely with what you eat. However, for optimal health, you should balance your intake of these two fatty acids: **omega-3** (alpha-linolenic, EPA, and DHA) and **omega-6** (linoleic), both of which are polyunsaturated fats. Good sources of omega-3s are dark green leafy vegetables, canola oil, flaxseed oil, soy, some nuts (e.g., walnuts), fish, and fish oils, while the omega-6s are more abundant in the corn, sunflower, peanut, and soy oils that constitute such food products as margarine, salad dressing, and cooking oils.

However, these days, eating healthier fats has been further complicated by farming practices. In organically raised meat (such as free-range chickens and grass-fed cows), the ratio of the two essential omegas is one to one, as it should be. In commercially raised animals, however, omega-6s are in excess, with the resulting meat often containing fourteen times more of them than of omega-3s. Fish is often touted as a "heart-healthy" food due to its usually high content of omega-3s, but farm-raised fish (which are very common now due to overfishing) have greater amounts of omega-6s than wild fish.

The problem with such an imbalance is that omega-6s are known to be pro-inflammatory, meaning that they may actually contribute to oxidative stress and potentially to heart disease, while omega-3 fatty acids are more anti-inflammatory and thus have the opposite effect. When you eat an excess of the pro-inflammatory type, it may actually accelerate your development of clogged arteries and a heart attack. Thus, most meat available these days may promote heart disease in more ways than one, and there is no easy solution other than to avoid eating much of it.

Avoid saturated and trans fats

Conversely, less-healthy saturated and trans fats found in dairy products, meat, partially or fully hydrogenated oils, and highly processed foods increase your levels of insulin resistance, thus making your diabetes control more difficult. You would do well to embrace dairy products with a lower fat content. As a recent twelve-week study showed, people who ate yogurt daily while on a diet lost 22 percent more weight (an average of 14 pounds), 66 percent more body fat, and 81 percent more stomach fat than those who did not eat yogurt. It is believed that the calcium found in dairy products such as yogurt actually increases your fat utilization and prevents the absorption of some of the fat in foods you eat. Choose low- or nonfat yogurt with artificial sweeteners for the best BG results.

Many unhealthy fats may be added to processed foods that you eat, and reading food labels is still the best way to find out if a product contains them. Fats, like added sugars, can be disguised in a number of forms, including palm, coconut, or palm kernel oil; mono- and diglycerides; stearate; palmitate; lard; vegetable shortening; and hydrogenated or partially hydrogenated oils. Various types of liquid oils, including corn, safflower, soybean, peanut, olive, and canola, are often collectively referred to as vegetable oils. The fats that are best for your heart and your diabetes are high in monounsaturated fatty acids, such as olive, macadamia nut, and canola oils; or in mostly polyunsaturated fats such as peanut oil that are typically liquid at room temperature. Oils that are more damaging to your coronary arteries and glycemic control are usually solid or semisolid at room temperature, such as saturated fats found in meat, dairy, the "tropical oils," and trans fats created when manufacturers hydrogenate or partially hydrogenate liquid oils to alter their texture.

TIP
28
NO MATTER YOUR WEIGHT

A HIGH intake of saturated and trans fats can contribute to the development of insulin resistance as much as added sugars and high-GI carbohydrates can. Try to cut down on your intake of all of these by eating more foods in their natural state, such as high-fiber fruits, vegetables, and legumes.

Lose some of the cholesterol, too

It is also smart to choose foods that limit your intake of cholesterol, which—along with saturated and trans fats—is still considered a culprit in the development of heart disease. Your body does use a certain amount of cholesterol—a waxy, fat-like substance that is an important component of cells and hormones. However, your liver manufactures about 70 percent of the cholesterol found in your blood and is capable of making more if you don't eat enough of it. Therefore, your maximal intake should not exceed 300 milligrams (mg) per day (or no more than 100 mg per 1,000 calories eaten). Cholesterol is present in all animal products, including meat, poultry, shellfish, fish, eggs, and dairy. The cholesterol in eggs is no longer believed to be quite as unhealthy as it once was, but since eggs contain almost 300 mg per egg yolk, it's easy to go overboard if you eat more than one egg at a time. The good news is that cholesterol is not found in any plant foods, including grains, vegetables, fruits, nuts, or legumes.

Cholesterol itself is not known to directly decrease the action of insulin, but if you already have some degree of insulin resistance, consuming foods high in cholesterol, which are typically also high in fat, can lead to an increase in your circulating blood fats (triglycerides, in particular) and contribute to the formation of LDL cholesterol. When LDL becomes oxidized, as it often does when your BG levels are poorly controlled, it has the potential to be even more damaging to your arteries. If LDL cholesterol is the "bad" cholesterol, HDL is the "good" cholesterol. Physical activity has a greater effect on your levels of HDL; a high level of regular activity elevates HDL levels, while a sedentary state lowers them. Diabetic men on low-GI diets have experienced improvements in both types of cholesterol (meaning that their LDL decreased while their HDL went up), which is another reason to consider following such a plan.

Eat more and weigh less

The best part of a high-fiber, unrefined diet is that you can eat more *and* weigh less. The calorie density of foods—more so than the amount you eat or even the overall fat content—contributes most to weight gain. To lose weight, you don't necessarily have to cut back on how much you eat if you simply eat "bigger" foods—that is, those that are bulked up by fiber and water, making them less calorie dense. Broth-based soups are generally lower in calories because of their high water (and usually vegetable) content (the sodium content can be high, though), and people who eat more of such soups usually have a lower body weight for their size. Even whipped foods may fill you up better because of their additional air content. Other high-volume foods include most vegetables, whole fruits, air-popped popcorn, and lettuce-based salads (with modest amounts of salad dressing).

Regardless of the calorie content of what you eat, your hunger will be best satisfied by eating the volume of food that your stomach is used to. So, you can trick yourself into eating fewer calories even when eating the same volume—for example, if you start your meal with a salad containing three cups of lettuce and vegetables and use a low-calorie salad dressing, you will eat an average of 12 percent fewer calories for any meal. If you have a salad with your spaghetti dinner, the salad alone would reduce your intake by 80 calories for a meal with the exact same volume. Although such small reductions may not seem like much, you would end up saving 560 calories in a week, about 2,300 a month, and 29,000 in a year—the equivalent of about eight pounds of body fat— just by adding a salad to your dinner and eating slightly less pasta. You eat the same volume of food, and you aren't left feeling hungry.

TIP
29

———————— **NO MATTER YOUR WEIGHT** ————————

MANY DIETS fail because eating a smaller volume of food than you are used to means you're hungry more often. A simple way to keep up the food volume and still lose weight is to include salads and more vegetables with your lunch and dinner. You can eat *more* of these foods and still end up weighing *less*.

Become a grazer

Speaking of hunger, there are other ways to avoid it that can also help you maintain or lose weight. Eating less at one sitting but more frequently is the best route to follow, particularly when you're trying to keep outpacing the ability of your beta cells to release insulin. In one study, overweight men were found to consume fewer calories when given the same total amount of food as several smaller meals instead of as a single, larger one. If you become a "grazer," or someone who eats small meals and snacks throughout the day, you'll typically end up leaner than someone who eats less often, even if you're eating an equivalent number of calories. Eating four to six smaller meals throughout the day may keep your metabolic rate at a higher level, thus increasing your overall energy expenditure for each day. By not becoming ravenously hungry between meals, you will also be less likely to overeat.

Always eat your breakfast . . . and lunch and dinner

In a similar vein, the timing of your meals can affect your body weight and overall health. So can skipping them. Breakfast is more important than you may realize as it serves to "break" your overnight fast, effectively kicking your fasting metabolism into a higher gear and lowering levels of hormones (like cortisol) that increase insulin resistance. Conversely, skipping your first meal sustains your fast and keeps your body in an energy-conserving mode (meaning you expend fewer calories until you eat), and meaning your body will likely remain less responsive to insulin. Healthy women who eat breakfast are more insulin sensitive throughout the day than women who skip it, and breakfast abstainers also consume a larger number of calories over the course of the day in spite of not consuming breakfast calories. In fact, people who eat breakfast tend to be leaner than people who skip it, and skipping breakfast increases your risk for developing type 2 diabetes (if you don't already have it).

You should never allow yourself to become overly hungry by skipping any meal, as doing so almost always results in overeating at later meals. Because your body's use of calories at any one time is limited, and the rest go into storage, eating most of your calories later in the day will generally cause you to become more overweight. Excess calories eaten at dinner or later are then stored as fat, which is done even more effectively in the evening when you're likely to be less active and then asleep. Sleeping results in your lowest level of energy expenditure of the day and allows for optimum fat and energy storage. If you skip breakfast (and possibly lunch) and save your main calorie consumption for dinner, you'll end up with higher levels of body fat for all of these reasons *and* have a greater risk of developing type 2 diabetes, despite having passed up a meal or two during the day.

A cup of coffee to go—or forgo?

Are you one of those people who can't survive without your daily caffeine fix? Recent studies declaring that coffee consumption lowers your risk of developing diabetes made headlines—and possibly made your heart soar with hope. Caffeine has no calories, and it actually stimulates your metabolism somewhat, so why shouldn't you have regular coffee with breakfast, as well as diet colas, iced tea, and other caffeinated drinks throughout the day? Well, because, according to even more recent research, rather than improving your chances of avoiding diabetes, caffeine causes your insulin to work less effectively—regardless of your body weight or exercise status. In lean, obese, and type 2 diabetic people equally, caffeine ingestion equivalent to two to three eight-ounce cups of coffee (5 milligrams per kilogram of body weight) reduces their insulin sensitivity by about one-third, and the caffeine-induced decrement is still present even if they undergo three months of moderate aerobic exercise training. Thus, you may want to think twice before loading up on a super-sized coffee to go (particularly if you are drinking it in place of breakfast).

Is healthier eating possible in a fast-food world?

More often than not, finding healthy snacks and meals on the run is difficult at best. In convenience markets, most of the snacks and foods available are filled with too much sugar, fat, and/or sodium. Fast-food fare also typically consists of high-fat and high-GI, calorie-dense, nutrient-poor choices, and food eaten in more formal dining settings (sit-down restaurants) is typically higher in fat than home-cooked versions. In addition, portion sizes count when you're trying to eat more nutritiously, and the oversized portions of typical ready-to-eat foods contribute vastly to our caloric intake. Portions at restaurants have also been increasing steadily over the past several decades, with supersized "value" menus plentiful and inexpensive.

It should come as no surprise, then, that if you eat out at restaurants frequently, you're likely to be more overweight than if you make a habit of eating home-cooked meals. Unfortunately, more and more people are eating on the run, and Americans now eat out for one meal out of three (as compared with one in twenty three decades ago). Most of us nowadays live fast-paced, hectic lives—working long hours, spending time commuting to and from work, chauffeuring our kids to their next activity. As a result, more of us eat on the run, and eating out makes us fatter and more prone to developing diabetes (or to having poorly controlled BG levels if we already have diabetes).

The abundance of buffet-style meals, such as all-you-can-eat pizza parlors, Chinese buffets, steakhouses, and other restaurants, definitely has not helped the situation. Invariably, you'll end up eating more than you need when you've paid for an unlimited amount of food and you're trying to get your money's worth. Moreover, when you eat in most fast-food restaurants, it's almost impossible to feel satiated without overloading on calories due to the food's high calorie density and low bulk. The lack of vegetables, salad, or fresh fruit, particularly that have not been doctored with extra butter, oil, dressing, or whipped cream, only compounds the problem. The higher GI value of the meal may also cause you to feel hungrier in the long run, even though you have eaten an excessive number of calories. I personally have yet to find an effective way to eat a buffet meal without having trouble controlling my BG levels for hours afterward, even if I go heavy on the salads and vegetables.

TIP
30

NO MATTER YOUR WEIGHT

IF YOU eat at fast-food restaurants at least twice a week, you may end up gaining an extra 10 pounds a year and experience a twofold increase in your insulin resistance compared with people who eat fast food less than once a week. If you have prediabetes or diabetes, you certainly don't want to add to your insulin resistance, so make a concerted effort to reduce the number of times you eat fast food per week.

The real deal on lighter, healthier meals

But what about the "lighter" menu items offered at some fast-food chains? Unfortunately, the motto of most of this healthier fare is (or should be), "Here today . . . gone tomorrow." For example, in the summer of 2004, McDonald's launched—then dropped—its Go Active Happy Meals for adults. These meals featured an entrée salad, bottled water, and a pedometer. (Who can blame them, really? How many pedometers can one person really use?) Similarly, Burger King got rid of its Lite Combo Meals, which offered chicken sandwiches with a side salad and bottled water. To its credit, though, the Wendy's restaurant chain has plans for a fresh-fruit bowl containing pineapple, cantaloupe, honeydew melon, and red grapes, offered with or without low-fat strawberry yogurt.

One good change has come about, though: salads at many fast-food restaurants finally contain something other than nutrition-lacking iceberg lettuce. For instance, Burger King's Tendercrisp garden salads now offer more nutrients and fiber from romaine lettuce, carrots, red onions, cucumbers, and grape tomatoes. However, the sodium and calorie content of the dressings is still quite high, so you would do better to use only half the package of salad dressing. Other restaurants have begun offering "heart healthy," "carb smart," and other such choices, but they may not always be the best choice for you. For example, some of the low-carbohydrate salads that you can order at dine-in fast-food restaurants like Ruby Tuesday have more calories and saturated fat than a steak and more sodium than a large order of French fries.

Trying to eat less fat is an easy way to reduce the calorie content of your food without changing the portion size, but simply reducing the energy density of your foods is likely a better solution. If you can, fill up on larger portions of foods lower in energy density, such as fruits and vegetables. These are admittedly still difficult to get on most fast-food menus, so you may have to eat meals at home more often or pack your own and bring them with you. With the limited number of healthier fast-food choices, some of which are not even available at all nationwide chains, it's still a struggle to eat well at such restaurants (which is why I don't eat in them at all).

The real cost of "value" meals

It is unlikely that all fast-food restaurants are going to do away with their "value" menus anytime soon to help us become healthier consumers, so you will need to educate yourself on your food intake. Simply cutting back your consumption of fast food is by far the best way to make your meals healthier. Besides, according to the latest estimates, for every 67 cents you save with a super-large "value" meal, you will spend an extra $1.57 on medical costs (for a net loss of 90 cents on each meal), so it's not much of a bargain in the end. However, even small food modifications may help, so cut back wherever you can to start, even if it's only to order a junior-size burger instead of a regular or oversized one.

A Mac attack or a heart attack?

If you have diabetes, there is another salient reason to limit your consumption of nutrition-poor fast foods: most health-care professionals already consider you to have the equivalent of heart disease, and consuming a typical fast-food meal can cause **endothelial dysfunction**, meaning that the blood flow through your arteries (which are lined with endothelial cells) is disturbed by eating these unhealthy foods. Thus, a fast-food diet can contribute to your arterial plaque formation even without any change in your cholesterol levels.

A recent documentary film, *Super Size Me*, reported the weight gain and health decline of an investigative reporter who ate his every meal at McDonald's for one month. During that month, his body weight skyrocketed as did his cholesterol levels. Actually, it's possible to find damage to your blood vessels and elevations in your blood fats after just *one* fast-food breakfast consisting of an egg McMuffin, a sausage McMuffin, and two hash browns, even if you're a young, healthy male in your twenties (the biggest consumers of fast food). Just imagine how much more endothelial damage you may be experiencing with such meals, or even worse ones like the Hardee's 1,400-calorie Monster Thickburger or Burger King's 1,000-calorie Double Whopper with cheese, given that your diabetes already makes you more prone to such deadly changes.

An alternate—the polymeal?

Some researchers are now advocating the "**polymeal**" to eliminate heart disease. The polymeal would replace the "polypill" (a combination of prescribed medications, all of which have potential side effects), and the take-home message of this new diet is that pharmacological methods are not the only, or even the best, way to reduce your heart disease risk factors, such as elevated blood fats and cholesterol, BG, and hypertension, or even your risk of developing diabetes in the first place. In fact, this new diet may be able to cut your risk of developing heart disease by 76 percent.

Interestingly, the polymeal plan advocates consumption of about 5 ounces of wine (preferably red) per day (to induce a 32 percent reduction in heart disease risk), 3 to 4 ounces of dark chocolate a day (a 21 percent reduction), about 4 ounces of fish four times a week (a 14 percent reduction—but watch your mercury intake), 13 ounces of fruits and vegetables daily (a 21 percent decrease), one-tenth of an ounce of garlic daily (a 25 percent drop), and at least 2 ounces of almonds a day (a 12.5 percent reduction), with a combined 63 to 84 percent (76 percent average) lower risk of cardiovascular problems—which is as good as or better than what you can achieve with a polypill. The scientific evidence to support these consumables' purported health benefits is discussed in the following section.

Alcohol. Many studies have been conducted on the ability of an alcoholic drink or two a day to increase your levels of HDL cholesterol and reduce your risk of heart disease. A recent meta-analysis (examining the results of fifteen research studies) determined that moderate alcohol consumption actually decreases your chances of developing type 2 diabetes by about 30 percent. Of course, "moderate" is the key word. People who drink 48 or more grams of alcohol daily do not decrease their diabetes risk. (A standard drink in the United States or Canada contains about 12 grams of alcohol, compared with 10 grams in Europe and Australia and 21 grams in Japan.) People who drink at least 6 grams per day (about half a glass of wine in the United States) actually have a lower diabetes risk than teetotalers. Keep in mind, though, that alcohol contains 7 calories per gram, which makes its calorie content closer to fat (which has 9 calories per gram) than carbohydrate or protein (both of which contain 4 calories per gram). Also, spreading your weekly alcohol consumption out evenly—such as consuming one drink per day instead of saving all seven for the weekend—is much more effective in reducing your risk.

Dark chocolate. Similarly, the effects of dark chocolate continue to be proven again and again, thanks to certain phytonutrients, in particular the flavanols and procyanidins contained in it (but not contained in white chocolate). Flavanols may protect your heart and blood vessels with their antioxidant properties and by increasing your blood flow by releasing more of a compound called "nitric oxide." It deeply influences your insulin-stimulated BG use and vascular tone, resulting in significant improvements in both insulin sensitivity and blood pressure when 100 grams of dark chocolate are consumed daily for fifteen days, as they were in healthy volunteers in a recent study. Dark chocolate appears to cause immediate dilation of small- and medium-sized blood vessels around your body, improving blood flow to all parts of it.

Fish. The health benefits of fish are also well proven. The omega-3 fatty acids found in fish, especially in species such as wild salmon, mackerel, lake trout, herring, and sardines, which have high levels, protect you against the development of cardiovascular disease. Be careful about consuming too much of fish that contain higher levels of mercury, though, including shark, swordfish, king mackerel, and tilefish. Five of the most commonly eaten fish that are low in mercury are shrimp, canned light tuna, salmon, pollack, and catfish. Albacore ("white") tuna has more mercury than canned light tuna, though, so you should eat six or fewer ounces of albacore tuna per week.

Alternate polymeals. A study recently conducted in Finland reached slightly different conclusions about what's best to eat for diabetes prevention. People who had higher intakes of green vegetables, fruit and berries, oil and margarine, and poultry had a reduced risk of developing type 2 diabetes. These conclusions agree with the concepts of healthier eating that we have discussed in this step, with the possible exception of poultry (unless it's lean). What their results really tell us, though, is that there is likely more than one combination of foods with healthy effects.

Similarly, people who eat a "Mediterranean-style" diet—rich in vegetables, fruits, nuts, legumes, whole grains, fish, and fats that come from plants, such as olive oil—also have a significantly reduced risk of dying from disease, especially heart disease and cancer, than anyone consuming less of these healthful foods and eating more saturated fat, meat, poultry, and full-fat dairy products. In a recent study of more than twenty-two thousand healthy people living in Greece, the group with the lowest mortality consumed about a pound of vegetables and nearly a pound of fruit daily. They also ate whole-grain bread, cereal, and pasta, but only in moderate amounts—moderation is the key—preferring instead to get many of their carbohydrates from fruit and vegetables. They also used olive oil in place of other fats, rather than in addition to them (or else they would likely have gained weight). Finally, the lowest mortality was also paired with drinking moderate amounts of alcohol: about a glass of wine a day for women, two glasses for men. Not surprisingly, their level of physical activity also made a difference in their risk of dying. The most physically active Greeks in the study—who exercised vigorously an hour daily (or did the equivalent of moderate walking for three hours a day)—had a 28 percent lower mortality rate than those who exercised less.

Polymeal versus polypill. Regardless of your current diet, given the choice between taking a "polypill" containing various medications to prevent or control diabetes, heart disease, or other health problems, and consuming a health-promoting "polymeal," hopefully you now realize that it's always better to achieve improved health the natural (nonpharmaceutical) way.

THE BOTTOM LINE ON STEP 4
Adopt an Optimal Eating Plan

▶ The composition of carbohydrate, fat, and protein that you eat is not nearly as important as limiting your intake of particular foods that affect your BG balance.

▶ Use the concepts of glycemic index and load to guide you to better food choices.

▶ Try to consume at least 50 grams of dietary fiber daily.

▶ Stick with natural foods high in fiber, phytonutrients, and nutrition.

▶ Eat a wide variety of colorful fruits and vegetables, which have more antioxidant power.

▶ Limit your intake of refined carbohydrates, added sugars, and unhealthy fats.

▶ Eat less-calorie-dense foods (but more of them) to avoid weight gain.

▶ Become a grazer, eating smaller meals but never skipping them altogether.

▶ Limit your caffeine intake, as it is likely to decrease your insulin action.

▶ Steer clear of most fast-food restaurants, as eating out at them frequently will likely cause you to gain weight and become more insulin resistant.

▶ Try the polymeal approach for balanced, healthy eating.

It should now be obvious to you that to reach your goal of diabetes fitness, you still have to pay some attention to what you eat—even though hopefully you aren't going to be going on any more fad diets.

Making small changes in your food and beverage intake will pay out big rewards, and it is truly worth making the effort to improve your nutritional status.

DIABETES FITNESS PLAN STEP 4
in a Nutshell

OPTIMAL EATING is just as vital to diabetes fitness as physical activity, as the two work in concert. Stick with natural, colorful, high-fiber, low-GI foods and smaller portions to control your diabetes and your body weight.

STEP 5

Get Emotionally Fit

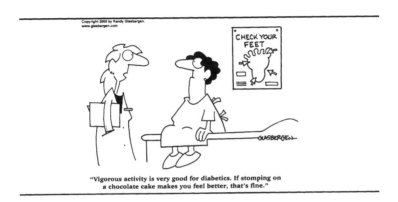

"Vigorous activity is very good for diabetics. If stomping on a chocolate cake makes you feel better, that's fine."

HAS DIABETES OR your weight got you down? Having a chronic health problem presents a special set of emotional challenges unlike any other. You may have taken on your health condition as a personal challenge, and vowed to do whatever is necessary to control it to the fullest extent possible. While such a proactive stance is generally helpful from a control standpoint, it can also lead you to become somewhat obsessive about your health and your daily care regimens—which may not be psychologically healthy and may even be counterproductive.

You may have responded in the opposite manner, however, acting at least initially as though your disease doesn't exist. This is the more common approach. You may have decided to ignore your health-care plan, forgo taking your prescribed medications, and disregard dietary and other recommendations that can immeasurably improve your health status (although, since you're reading this book, you've likely decided on some version of the former stance). As you now know, ignorance is *not* bliss when it comes to diabetes or prediabetes, since you can't prevent or control them and their related health complications without making a concerted effort. In the case of diabetes, what you don't know *can* kill you.

Here's a news bulletin for you about your emotional health: regular exercise, not dieting, is the answer to all of your diabetes blues. Despite all of the potentially negative psychological effects of dealing with chronic health problems such as obesity and diabetes, exercise has the ability to relieve all of your worst emotional symptoms and to enhance your mood. The next step to diabetes fitness, discussed in the sections that follow, will show you how.

Emotional concerns arising from diabetes or your weight

Regardless of how you responded to your diagnosis of type 2 diabetes (and possibly other concurrent health conditions), you likely have special emotional concerns that often arise in anyone dealing with an "incurable," chronic health condition. No one feels good about being treated as physically inferior or being shunned by others for being overweight or for having diabetes. It's a reality for many people, though; the ADA recently organized a campaign to sponsor federal legislation to keep you from being discriminated against in the workplace because of your diabetes (which only can mean that it's happening). Diabetes is a less obvious condition than being overweight. Being denigrated, maligned, or discriminated against because of your body weight alone can easily play into and worsen any feelings of low self-esteem that you may already be having.

TIP

31

NO MATTER YOUR WEIGHT

WHILE DIABETES may be essentially "invisible" to others, being overweight (as most people with type 2 diabetes are) is clearly visible. Either condition, though—whether visible to your family, friends, and others or not—can wreak havoc on your emotional health.

Don't let diabetes or your weight get you down

How can you tell if you're depressed? True clinical depression is much different than the occasional bout of "the blues" that everyone experiences from time to time, especially when bad things happen. Depression lasts much longer, often going on for months without any lasting relief. When you are depressed, you may feel sad and hopeless, and you may lose interest in things you normally enjoy. You may also eat or sleep much more or less than usual, have very low energy levels, have trouble concentrating, and feel really bad about yourself.

In the United States, about one adult in ten has **major depressive disorder**—the most serious form of depression—but it is more than twice as common among people with diabetes. In fact, researchers estimate that almost half of all people with diabetes have either major or milder forms of depression. While the odds of experiencing major depression are more than double if you have diabetes, it may be even greater if you have other health problems as well. The coexistence of heart disease, chronic arthritis, and strokes in particular are associated with an increased chance of major depression. All types of depressive disorders can seriously affect your ability to care for and control your health, often by decreasing your commitment to exercising regularly and/or following an appropriate diet.

A recent study conducted in Finland found a positive relationship between increasing insulin resistance and more severe depressive symptoms; what was really surprising was that it appears that this association is already present if you have impaired glucose tolerance, *before* the appearance of type 2 diabetes. Thus, it appears that prediabetes may also make you more prone to depression. Some researchers believe that depression itself may be contributing to the development of diabetes, rather than the other way around—another overwhelming reason to control not just diabetes, but also prediabetes.

Too much cortisol?

The link among all of these health conditions and depression is likely excessive levels of cortisol, which is released by your body in response to any type of physical or emotional stress. Depressed individuals have higher circulating levels of cortisol, and people with elevated levels of this natural hormone are not only more insulin resistant, but are also more likely to have depressed immune systems, making them more likely to get sick. Excess levels of cortisol are also at least partially responsible for low-level systemic inflammation, which may be the link between depression and the development of type 2 diabetes.

Your cortisol levels can also rise when your BG levels are not well controlled, serving only to exacerbate your already elevated sugars by making the insulin that your body does produce less effective and causing your pancreatic beta cells to work overtime to make even more insulin. It's a vicious cycle that is best broken by regular physical activity. Once you begin to exercise, your energy levels are likely to rise and your physical health to improve. Feeling better physically will in turn lessen your depressive thought patterns.

Yo-yo dieters, beware

We already discussed the fact that yo-yo dieters are generally worse off in the long run, but now there's another reason to avoid doing the "weight off, weight back on" routine: repeated failed attempts at sustained weight loss are not only potentially physically detrimental, but also more damaging to your emotional health. The medical community now advocates acquiring new behaviors that you can control, such as improving the quality of the food you consume and the amount and type of physical activity that you do, rather than focusing on attaining an "ideal" body weight or losing a certain number of pounds—which is certainly going to be a losing battle over the long haul for the vast majority of people.

TIP
32
NO MATTER YOUR WEIGHT

IT HAS been known for decades that if you are overweight or obese, you will not likely be able to stay on a diet. If you do manage to stick with it, you probably won't lose that much weight, and even if you are one of the lucky few who manage to lose a large amount, you'll eventually regain it. In short, dieting is an unnatural behavior that can easily result in an increased preoccupation with food, depression, and patterns of **disordered eating**.

The mind-body connection

Another reason to try to enhance and uplift your mood is the very well documented, but poorly understood, **mind-body connection**. Physical health and mental health are undeniably interrelated, and each affects the other; accordingly, your physical well-being often can't be improved if your psychological problems haven't been adequately addressed. Depression is an illness affecting both your mind and your body. When in a depressed state, you may feel sluggish, lethargic, apathetic toward your self-care, or downright uninterested in everything. Is it any wonder that it's difficult to manage your diabetes and stay healthy when you're depressed? While it's bad enough that diabetes makes you more prone to depression, even more alarming is the fact that depression apparently increases the likelihood that you—but not your nondiabetic friends—will die in the next 10 years. Out of more than 500 people with diabetes in a recent study, the depressed ones had a 54 percent greater mortality rate than those without depression.

It's undoubtedly harder to comply with your health-care plan when you feel physically unwell. In addition to sluggishness caused by elevated BG levels, chronic pain—either from diabetic neuropathy or other causes—is common in people with diabetes, with as many as 60 percent of subjects in one study reporting having it. Chronic pain appears to be a major limiting factor in your compliance with basic diabetes self-care, such as regular exercise or taking medications, both of which are important for minimizing your potential for diabetes-related complications and for improving your mental health.

Does stress really cause gray hairs?

A recent study on mothers caring for children who had life-threatening diseases like cancer found an accelerated aging of the mothers' DNA, so you may actually be right if you believe that excessive or prolonged emotional stress can give you more gray hairs or drive you to an early grave. Stress has a major impact on your circulatory system, and it plays a significant role in susceptibility to, progress in, and outcome of cardiovascular disease.

Not all stress is bad, however—for example, temporary stress during an athletic event may improve your ability to perform both emotionally and physically—but emotional stress due to diabetes or other chronic illnesses is likely more detrimental than helpful. A case in point is the fact that any stress (even simply making it through the holiday season) can suppress your body's immune function and increase your likelihood of getting sick—even with the common cold—by increasing your cortisol levels. Compound that level of stress day after day by living with diabetes and throw depression into the mix, and it's easy to understand why people with diabetes need to learn how to control their stress levels before they further negatively affect their physical health.

Don't worry—be happy

The science of happiness is currently being studied, and although about 50 percent of your capacity to feel happy may be attributable to genetics (i.e., your inherited personality), the other half is up to you. New research indicates that being grateful for what you have and connecting with others socially are two of the most important factors not only in avoiding depression, but also in reaching a higher level of happiness, which is especially important in dealing with diabetes. Feelings of happiness can keep you from overstressing and from overindulging in "taboo" comfort foods that may raise your BG levels and make you feel guilty. In addition, enjoying a greater overall happiness level will likely lead you to better self-care, including adherence to your daily exercise plan. (A free happiness-assessment survey can be accessed online at www.reflectivehappiness.com.)

The main point to remember about happiness is that you have to find it for yourself. Engaging in negative thought patterns and dwelling on the bad things in your life are surefire ways to stay unhappy. You are the only one with the capacity to change your thoughts for the better. If you are feeling a negative emotion, acknowledge it, but then tell it to get lost by replacing it with a positive one. You have the power to change how you view any situation or occurrence in your life, choosing to change it from a downer to an upper. For example, it would be easy for anyone with diabetes to feel depressed over the fact that it's currently an incurable condition. Alternately, wouldn't you end up feeling better about your diabetes and your life in general if you looked at all the tools at your disposal to control your BG levels and attempt to conquer it on your own? At least you'd be taking positive steps to control the things that you *can* influence and letting go of the things that you *can't*. Doing so will inevitably make you a much happier person.

Emotional fitness through physical activity

Personally, I have yet to decide whether my stress disappears after physical workouts because it actually enhances my mood, or if, at that point, I'm just too tired to care about my problems as much. In either case, it is well known that exercise is vitally important in alleviating your feelings of stress, anxiety, and depression. Everyone—people with and without chronic health conditions—can use regular exercise to relieve mild to moderate symptoms of depression and anxiety, as well as to improve mood and self-perceptions. If you're physically active, particularly if you're a woman (which already makes you more prone to depression than a man), you'll experience better mental and physical health and less depression than someone who is physically inactive.

Here's how exercise comes in as the best "medicine" once again. As I mentioned previously, becoming physically active can also positively affect your self-perceptions, benefiting your self-confidence, self-concept, and self-esteem. Especially for us women and girls, dissatisfaction with our bodies is associated with lower self-esteem. If you perceive yourself as fat and out of shape, you'll be particularly vulnerable to a negative self-image. We're all more and more susceptible to such bodily misperceptions because of television; for instance, overweight teens who spend more time watching soap operas, movies, music videos, and sports reportedly have an even greater bodily dissatisfaction and drive for thinness than those who don't. Exercise acts as "medicine" because it can improve your body shape and size and, consequently, raise your self-esteem and improve your bodily satisfaction, particularly if you're overweight. Not only can exercise improve your short-term mental state and mood, but you can also use it to increase your overall sense of well-being over the long haul.

TIP

33

———— **NO MATTER YOUR WEIGHT** ————

IF YOU perceive yourself as fat and out of shape, you will be more vulnerable to a negative self-image. Try exercising to improve your self-esteem. Even a low level of physical activity (e.g., exercising one to two times per week) can positively improve your mental health and attitudes about your physical state—not to mention your physical health itself.

Love those endorphins

One of the purported emotional benefits of exercise is related to the release of hormones in your brain called **endorphins**. These mood-enhancing hormones bind to your brain's natural receptors and are responsible for the so-called runner's high, which is described as a feeling of euphoria after you have been exercising for a while. Those of us who don't run call it our "second wind," or when we start feeling good enough to keep on exercising. Some people are positively addicted to this release of endorphins and need to get their daily dose.

Now there is another reason why exercise and endorphin release is so good for you: endorphins may actually improve your body's insulin action, thereby reversing or decreasing insulin resistance. In fact, it is now thought that endorphin release may be a major mechanism in the enhanced insulin sensitivity attributable to moderate exercise training. If that's the case, go for maximum endorphins on a daily basis, and as a side benefit, you will be less depressed and anxious and enjoy a greatly improved mood.

Try the RIB principle to relax

Another good idea is to use the time that you exercise to simultaneously work on your emotional health through relaxation techniques. Specifically, optimize your mental and physical health by following the **RIB principle**, where the R stands for relaxation, the I for imagination, and the B for breathing. Try to relax while you are exercising; let your troubles flow out of your body, punch the air with your fists to release your anger or anxiety, and consciously try to relax the tense muscles in your body. Next, use your imagination to visualize more blood flowing to parts of your body that need it (like your heart, muscles, and diabetic feet). Some studies have actually shown that people can enhance blood flow to their feet simply by visualizing more blood flowing to them— verifying that a very strong mind-body connection really exists. Finally, take slow, deep, and steady breaths and release them slowly as well. (Don't do this during heavy aerobic exercise, however; use the time during your warmup and cool-down periods instead for best results.) At any time during a workout take deeper breaths if you are feeling winded, as more oxygen is brought into your body during a deep breath than during a shallow one.

The effect of food on your mood

How many times have you found yourself eating out of boredom or because of stress, social pressure, or other reasons? Eating certain foods elicits the release of various brain hormones that can actually soothe your anxiety and depression—but only up to a point. Indulging in foods like chocolate to excess to enhance your mood can later leave you feeling guilty and depressed over the weight you may have gained or the resulting elevations in your BG level due to your binge. Moreover, emotional reactions like these can result in longer-term issues and a dysfunctional relationship with food. Research has also shown that eating sugar and consuming caffeine to alter your mood at best gives you a temporary emotional "high," which will more often than not be followed by a later "crash."

If you're looking for an emotional pick-me-up from your food, some consumables may have a more long-term positive effect. Among these better choices are foods high in omega-3 fatty acids (e.g., fish and many nuts), which are also good for the health of your cardiovascular system. Healthy carbohydrates like those found in whole fruits, replete with fiber, vitamins and minerals, and phytonutrients, also have a soothing effect—in moderation, of course. For the sake of your emotional health and your diabetes, try to avoid bingeing on highly refined carbohydrates. Also focus on taking in enough of the B vitamins (discussed more fully in the next step), particularly folate, niacin, B_6, and B_{12}, which are found in abundance in high-fiber carbohydrate foods such as legumes. Drinking plenty of water or other noncaloric, noncaffeinated fluids also helps, as does making sure that you eat a healthy breakfast every morning.

Food, lifestyle, and your mental ability

Not only can your choice of foods affect your emotions, it can also affect your mental capacity to reason, remember, and function in general. For years, foods such as blueberries have been studied to determine if you're less likely to develop either **dementia** or **Alzheimer's disease** if you consume more of them. Researchers have concluded that your diet does play a role in preserving your mental function as you age, but that so do other health conditions.

If you are overweight now or were overweight or obese in middle age, you have an increased risk of developing dementia at some point in your life. Moreover, by having insulin resistance and diabetes, you also run a much higher risk of experiencing mental decline due to either Alzheimer's or other forms of dementia. One potential cause is plaque formation in the arteries that feed your brain; strokes, which are usually the result of brain ischemia caused by carotid artery blockage, are also a common complication of diabetes and one that can dramatically alter your cognitive abilities. However, there also appears to be a link between declining nerve function in your brain, systemic inflammation, and oxidative damage caused by **free radicals** that is just beginning to be better understood. Have you caught on to the recurring theme of inflammation being associated with chronic diseases yet?

Fight back by keeping your mind active

The good news is that you can prevent some of this potential loss of memory and mental functioning over time. All you need to do is eat better, exercise more, control your diabetes, smoke less, and—equally important—frequently exercise your mind with challenging endeavors. Whether that means that you finally take that class to learn Italian, hit the crossword puzzles hard, enter a chess competition, practice memory exercises, burn up the dance floor during dance lessons, or do daily mental "gymnastics" of your choosing to challenge your brain, the positive effects will be the same. It's now clear that if you're mentally active throughout your lifetime, you will be significantly less likely to suffer from a decline in your mental capacity in your later years. In general, people who are more educated, have more intellectually challenging jobs, and engage in more mentally stimulating activities, such as attending lectures and plays, reading, playing chess, and doing hobbies, are much less likely to develop Alzheimer's and other forms of dementia. Even if you have the feeling your mental processes are already on the decline, you can still reverse the trend. Elderly people who go through training to sharpen their wits, for example, score much better on thinking tests for years afterward, and even the minds of younger people who drill their memories seem to work more efficiently.

Scientists suspect that a lifetime of thinking a lot may create a cognitive reserve, a reservoir of brain power that you can draw upon even if you suffer a damaging silent stroke or protein deposits, which are the hallmarks of Alzheimer's. You will likely benefit most from engaging in a rich diversity of stimulating activities. New experiences may be far more important than repeating the same task over and over; try combining mental stimulation with social interaction for the greatest benefits. Most of all, you should enjoy the activities that you choose to take part in, because stress and other negative emotions appear to be harmful to your mental abilities (not to mention your BG control). Even relaxation techniques may benefit your mental functioning for that reason.

Dieting is the origin of most unhealthy relationships with food

We all have to eat. As I mentioned previously, though, if you repeatedly attempt and fail at dieting, you're much more likely to develop abnormal or unhealthy emotions toward food. Not surprisingly, then, most disordered eating is considered a mental health issue rather than a food and dieting issue. The problem is widespread: half a million people in the United States are battling disordered eating at any given time. Adults suffering from such disorders range from the underweight to the morbidly obese, but they include many people of normal weight, too.

Thankfully, more and more health and nutrition professionals are realizing that dieting is not a viable long-term solution to weight control for most people. They're finally starting to realize that forced dieting will only encourage you to develop dysfunctional eating habits and force you to obsess about your food and body weight rather than putting your focus where it should be: on achieving and maintaining good health and preventing further weight gain. Disordered eating, along with the more well-defined eating disorders, is triggered by a number of factors, the most common being low self-esteem, poor body image, perfectionist attitudes, stress, and anxiety.

TIP

34

―――――― **NO MATTER YOUR WEIGHT** ――――――

IF YOU are overweight and have diabetes, you are much more likely to have some form of disordered eating given that you're likely struggling to gain or maintain control over both your body weight and your BG levels. Your excess body weight is not at the core of your disordered eating, though, and should not be the focus of your treatment. Seek out assistance to deal with your altered emotional relationship with food, and your diabetes control will naturally follow.

How dysfunctional attitudes toward food take root

Where do we pick up the ideas that trigger such dysfunctional emotional attitudes and behaviors when it comes to our health, body weight, and nourishment? The strongest pressures come from *outside* and may include family, peer, and other pressures. When we're young and impressionable, it is common for us to internalize the attitudes of people we love and idolize, like our parents, but parental attitudes are far from being the only influences operating on us. Friends and peers are major influences on our views on body image and food—not to mention cultural influences. Eating an abundance of frequently unhealthy food at family gatherings is both common and expected among Americans. Look at the attitudes toward food that are portrayed on TV, as well. The *Drew Carey Show* is just one of many shows that stereotype obese characters as lowlifes with appalling eating habits and unhealthy relationships. Whenever something goes wrong, at least one character responds by grabbing something unhealthy to eat or drink, thus reinforcing the idea that using food for comfort or as a coping mechanism is normal and expected. Is it any wonder, then, that dysfunctional attitudes toward food are so prevalent in today's society?

How do you know if you have an eating disorder?

The mental health community has come up with specific definitions for four conditions that fall under the general heading of eating disorders: **anorexia nervosa**, **bulimia nervosa**, binge-eating disorder, and "eating disorder not otherwise specified" (or, more simply put, "dysfunctional eating"). A full discussion of these disorders is beyond the scope of this book, but readers are referred to the "bible" of the mental health profession, the *Diagnostic and Statistical Manual of Mental Disorders*, as well as ANRED (Anorexia Nervosa and Related Eating Disorders, Inc., accessed online at www.anred.com), as potential places to start looking for more information.

Not all eating disorders are as severe or as easily identified as anorexia (self-starvation) and bulimia (binge-purge disorder), and many are simply less obvious combinations of some or all of them. For example, you may have stopped eating as much as usual or become much choosier about foods to self-impose a diet. You may, alternatively, have started eating in secret. If, on the other hand, you start eating more food after a full meal, you may be doing so out of sadness, boredom, depression, or other emotional reasons. Moreover, you may eat large amounts of pizza and fries or drink excessive amounts of beer and other alcoholic beverages at social gatherings when you know you really shouldn't, just because you don't want to stand out. Finally, elevated BG itself creates a drive to eat that has nothing to do with true hunger.

Dealing with abnormal eating

How do you know when you are harming your health with abnormal eating patterns? We all go through phases when our eating habits change—the key is how often they change. If you are regularly eating more than necessary (or less, for that matter), then there is probably something amiss with your emotional state that could negatively affect your physical health if not remedied, especially if you have diabetes.

Realistically, though, you will not reverse the progress of eating disorders easily on your own. If you feel uncomfortable talking with a friend or relative about your problem, consult with a health-care professional specializing in diabetes care and/or eating disorders. In any way possible, give yourself as much love and understanding as you can so that your motivation to take better care of the only body you have to live in will strengthen and prevail.

The importance of impulse control

If you are offered some pleasantly aromatic chocolate chip cookies right out of the oven, what are the chances that you will be able to pass on eating one just because you think you should? The internal battle is between desire and self-control, between immediate gratification and delay. We all have to deal with such battles on a daily basis. In the United States today, our society is totally focused on satisfying our every desire—and doing it *now*. Resisting impulse, however, is the root of all emotional self-control, and changing your health habits for the better depends on your ability to be more focused on your future health benefits than on your immediate desires. In order to eradicate type 2 diabetes in young and old alike, our biggest battle is to learn both individually and as a society to stop gratifying and "supersizing" our immediate desires.

Does this need for preventive health habits mean that if you eat even one cookie, all is lost? Of course not. Eating one aromatic cookie slowly and savoring every nibble is certainly allowed—in fact, you may be more likely to eat just that one since you won't be obsessing about not getting to eat any. What, however, if you overindulge and eat the whole plateful of cookies? What then? Does this mean that all hope for moderate eating is lost? Thankfully, you don't need to give up hope. Although binge-eating disorders are more prevalent in diabetic individuals, breaking your abstinence from cookies with overindulgence is considered akin to "falling off the wagon" with drug or alcohol abuse. Don't beat yourself up with your guilt to the point of losing all motivation to resume your more healthful regimens as soon as possible. As long as you get back on the better nutrition wagon after the "fall," your good intentions will not have been for naught.

TIP

35

NO MATTER YOUR WEIGHT

COMPLETE ABSTINENCE from beloved treats and other culinary temptations is *not* the best way to approach lifetime eating changes. Instead, allow yourself to have small amounts of the foods that you really enjoy, and take your time eating them to maximize your enjoyment.

Moderation, not abstinence, is the key

If you've ever dieted, you know that it's easy to break down and end up gorging on forbidden treats, especially if you're having a bad day. To maintain a lifelong, healthy meal plan as advocated by this book, you don't need to completely abstain from any food. In fact, you can eat anything your heart desires . . . with one catch: you must learn to consume unhealthier foods *in moderation.*

What constitutes moderation, you ask? That is an extremely relevant (and often difficult) question. Rest assured that eating a dozen chocolate chip cookies at one sitting is not moderate—nor is consuming half a dozen. Moderation would likely be eating no more than one to two cookies (depending on their size). So, if you actually eat only one (or two) of the tempting cookies just discussed, you have practiced impulse control and successfully achieved moderation. (Give yourself a pat on the back—*not* another cookie!) Your interpretation of moderation needs to be revisited occasionally to keep it honest. Practicing moderation does not mean you get to eat that one cookie repeatedly, i.e., eating just one cookie three to four times a day. A good rule of thumb is that if the item you are eating is a high-GI, high-GL food, you should limit your consumption of it to no more than one small serving per day.

Practice makes perfect

You can teach yourself to be moderate by practicing. If you're having a rich dessert, try serving yourself half of your normal amount on a smaller plate (to make it look larger) and take twice as long as usual to eat it. Believe it or not, it is really the first couple of bites that taste the best, and you will feel just as—or more—satisfied after eating the smaller quantity (not to mention less guilty) if you really enjoy it. Slower eating allows all of your senses to experience and enjoy the flavor, while allowing your stomach to register its fullness in conscious regions of your brain. Your stomach is communicating with your brain without your realizing it through stretch receptors that then make you conscious of feeling full.

Some other strategies can also help you learn how to eat more moderately. Not only should you eat desserts more slowly, but you should also slow down on finishing the rest of your meal. Make a conscious effort to push back from the table *before* you're stuffed to the gills. Stop eating when you are about 80 percent full (or at least leave a few bites on your plate), and, amazingly, you'll feel 100 percent satisfied after a short while (instead of stuffed). Drinking water or another fluid before a meal or starting with broth-based soups also has the ability to make you feel full before you eat as much. If you tend to wolf down your food, wait at least 10 minutes (preferably 15 to 20 minutes) after finishing your first (moderate) helping before going back for seconds. (Usually during that waiting period, your stomach miraculously begins to feel fuller as well.) Better yet, plan a light snack for two to three hours after your meal instead of stuffing yourself at any one time. If you fail to eat enough fruit or healthier foods during the day, your snack can consist of any unfinished veggies from dinner, complemented with fruit and low-fat yogurt, an apple and peanut butter, or some other combination of healthy foods.

TIP

36

NO MATTER YOUR WEIGHT

EATING MORE slowly (no matter what you are eating) results in your feeling full more quickly and thus in your eating less. Try this approach for all your meals and snacks and, despite eating less, you'll never leave the table hungry.

How to deal with "un-moderate" situations

As a society, we have practiced the opposite of moderation. In fact, we've all learned how to gorge ourselves on occasions revolving around feasting (which is practically all of them nowadays). However, I speak from experience when I tell you that it is utterly impossible for anyone with diabetes to balance BG levels in the short term when food intake is excessive at any one meal. You'll have to either practice developing your self-control or simply avoid tempting all-you-can-eat buffets, family-style restaurants, potluck dinners, holiday feasts, and other similar occasions, which are anything but moderate if you don't stop yourself from eating too much.

However, if you find yourself faced with a buffet-style meal you simply can't avoid, you can still fight back. The best idea is to consume a full plateful of salad (but go easy on the dressing) and vegetables first, wait at least 10 to 15 minutes, and then return for a second, smaller plateful of entrée "samples." Use smaller plates if they're available. Also, never go back for a third helping, be sure to eat slowly, drink plenty of water or noncaloric fluids during the meal, and try to stop eating well before you are completely stuffed. If you just have to have a dessert, take a half serving and eat it slowly to really enjoy it, as I described previously.

THE BOTTOM LINE ON STEP 5
Get Emotionally Fit

▶ It is likely that you have special emotional concerns from dealing with a chronic health condition like diabetes or excess body weight.

▶ Almost half of all people with diabetes have either major or milder forms of depression.

▶ Elevated levels of cortisol are associated with depression and diabetes.

▶ Your happiness is in your own hands, so adjust your thought patterns to take control over what you can influence.

▶ Physical fitness gives you a jump start on achieving emotional fitness.

▶ The release of brain endorphins with exercise enhances mood and decreases anxiety.

▶ Foods can affect your emotions and your mental capacity.

▶ Having diabetes increases your risk of developing Alzheimer's disease and dementia, but being physically active lowers it.

► Disordered eating is a common and treatable mental health condition often stemming from repeated attempts at dieting.

► Practicing moderation in eating, not complete abstinence from certain foods, is paramount in controlling your BG levels over the long haul.

Much of your success in making permanent lifestyle changes stems from your ability to love yourself enough to want to be as healthy as possible. You're living in the only body that you'll ever have. Make it your temple. Start by taking small steps toward better health, and then keep moving forward on that more positive emotional and physical path. With your stress and depression under better control, it will be easier for you to successfully follow through with the next step in achieving diabetes fitness—taking diabetic medications and supplements, which is fully discussed in the following section.

DIABETES FITNESS PLAN STEP 5
in a Nutshell

YOUR EMOTIONAL health is just as important as your physical health when it comes to effectively controlling your diabetes and preventing loss of quality of life from depression, dementia, or disordered eating. Physical activity can help you conquer them all.

STEP 6

Make the Most of Meds and Supplements

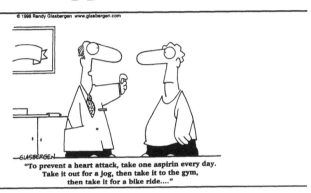

© 1998 Randy Glasbergen www.glasbergen.com

—GLASBERGEN—

"To prevent a heart attack, take one aspirin every day.
Take it out for a jog, then take it to the gym,
then take it for a bike ride...."

N O MATTER WHAT your diabetes treatment regimen consists of—exercise, dietary changes, oral diabetic medications, insulin, **nutritional supplements**, herbal remedies, and/or stress-reduction techniques—it must be able to effectively control your BG levels. Ideally, your glucose level should never go above 140 mg/dl, and your average BG level (over about a month) should result in a glycated hemoglobin (**HbA1c**) level of less than or equal to 7 percent to be considered truly effective. Thus, if exercise and diet alone aren't doing the job, you may need to consider your other options, particularly medication. Although your physician will decide which medication(s) you should try, a better understanding of what you're taking will make you able to determine for yourself if your medication regimen is really right for your unique body.

Will you also benefit from taking nutritional supplements such as chromium, vanadium, or cinnamon to increase your insulin sensitivity? The answer is that there is no way to know for certain until you have tried out the supplement. This step to achieving fitness with diabetes will tell you what you need to know about diabetic medications, supplements, and herbal remedies to achieve optimal BG control.

The third cornerstone in diabetes management

The medical community acknowledges three cornerstones in diabetes management. Although my bias is that becoming physically fit is the best way to manage your diabetes (hence, I would call exercise the first cornerstone), you should by now realize that optimal BG control includes paying adequate attention to your diet as well—making diet the second, but an equally important, management tool. Effective use of diabetic medications is considered the third cornerstone in diabetes management.

Anyone with type 1 diabetes already has to take daily doses of insulin, likely in multiple injections or infusions, but if you have type 2 diabetes, you may not be taking any prescribed medications. However, since type 2 diabetes is a progressive disease (meaning that your BG control may deteriorate over time as you continue to lose beta-cell function), an appropriate regimen of diabetic medications is likely to become equally imperative in your quest to become fit, successfully meet your BG targets, and prevent any further health complications.

For instance, you may have good BG control in the morning, but an excessive rise after meals, making certain medications more advantageous than others. Or perhaps your problem is high sugars first thing in the morning, although you do pretty well at other times of the day; you may benefit from a different diabetic medication. Or maybe you have tried them all, alone and in combination, and nothing seems to work well enough; your only remaining medical option may be to add in injections of supplemental insulin. No matter which medications you take, though, keep in mind that being physically active may very well eliminate your need for such medications or at least lower the dosages you need to take either immediately or down the road.

Oral diabetic medications

If you have been prescribed an oral diabetic medication (or more than one) to better control your diabetes and meet your glycemic goals, it comes from one of the classes of medications currently approved primarily to treat type 2 diabetes in the United States. Keep in mind that some prescribed medications are actually combinations of compounds from two different classes and, therefore, have the actions of both classes (e.g., Glucovance and Metaglip, which combine a **sulfonylurea** and a **biguanide**; and Avandamet, a combination of a "glitazone" and a biguanide). The approved medication classes are detailed in the table that follows.

Oral Diabetic Medications

CLASS OF DRUG	EXAMPLES (BRAND NAME)	MECHANISM OF ACTION(S)
Thiazolidenediones "Glitazones"	Avandia Actos	Increase insulin sensitivity of peripheral tissues, such as muscle
Biguanides	Glucophage, Glucophage XR, Riomet, Glumetza, metformin (generic)	Decrease liver glucose output; increase liver and muscle insulin sensitivity; no direct effect on beta cells
Sulfonylureas	Amaryl, DiaBeta, Diabinese, Glynase, Micronase	Promote insulin secretion from the beta cells of the pancreas; some may raise insulin sensitivity
Meglitinides/ Phenylalanine derivatives	Prandin, Starlix	Stimulate beta cells to increase insulin secretion, but only for a very short duration (unlike sulfonylureas)
Alpha-glucosidase inhibitors	Precose, Glyset	Work in intestines to slow digestion of some carbohydrates to control postmeal blood glucose peaks
Amylin*	Symlin	Works in combination with insulin to control glycemic spikes for three hours after meals
Incretins*	Byetta, liraglutide (generic)	Stimulate insulin release; inhibit the liver's release of glucose via glucagon; delay the emptying of food from the stomach

*Only available by injection at this time.

Thiazolidinediones. A group of **insulin sensitizers**, the **thiazolidinediones**, are most closely related in a physiological way to the insulin-sensitizing effects of physical activity. Although one drug from this class was taken off the market (Rezulin, for possibly causing liver damage), two other medications, Avandia and Actos, are being used without significant side effects. They improve insulin sensitivity, do not cause hypoglycemia, and can be taken once daily. While these medications have been found to occasionally cause fluid retention, Avandia in particular appears to improve blood flow and decrease the formation of plaque in coronary arteries. By improving cardiac function and exercise capacity—both of which are often low if you have diabetes—this medication may increase your ability to engage in physical activity. In addition to increasing your muscles' use of BG at rest, Avandia also doubles your body's responsiveness to circulating insulin during exercise.

Biguanides. A second class of drugs is the biguanides. **Metformin** is the generic name of the only compound in this class with FDA approval, but it is marketed under several different trade names, such as Glucophage and Glucophage XR. Its primary advantage over the sulfonylureas (e.g., DiaBeta and Glucotrol) is that it is not capable of inducing hypoglycemia when taken alone; rather, it exerts its effect by shutting down your liver's excessive production of glucose overnight, making it excellent for treating morning hyperglycemia, and it also improves the action of your insulin in both your liver and your muscles. It's also the only oral diabetic medication that promotes weight loss, which is another reason why it is so frequently prescribed by physicians; however, it only works in this capacity if you use shorter-acting Glucophage rather than one of the extended release forms (Glucophage XR or Glumetza). Finally, metformin appears to be somewhat protective of the heart compared with other diabetic medications.

Biguanides are not without potential side effects, though. Mild nausea and diarrhea are common if you use it, although taking it with meals generally decreases these symptoms. You may also be more tolerant of the sustained-release preparations. If you come down with an acute illness while taking it, you may have to discontinue it until you're well, as it may induce a state of lactic acidosis (where lactic acid builds up in your circulation). Another potentially negative aspect of metformin is that it can reverse ovulatory abnormalities found in some overweight women, leading to a greater risk of unplanned pregnancies in premenopausal women.

Meglitinides. Other possible medication regimens include **meglitinides**, Prandin or Starlix, which may have advantages for you if you eat sporadically. You can take these just when you eat to cause your pancreas to release enough insulin to cover any BG spikes. If you're one of those people who experiences large increases in your BG levels shortly after eating, you will definitely benefit the most from using one of these medications—as long as your beta cells still have the capacity to sufficiently increase their insulin production. They are also safe for use by pregnant women who are experiencing gestational diabetes during their pregnancy.

Alpha-glucosidase inhibitors. Another class of FDA-approved medications, **alpha-glucosidase inhibitors** control your glycemic spikes by slowing the absorption of carbohydrates from your stomach when you take them immediately before meals. Even pregnant women with gestational diabetes can safely use either Precose or Glyset, the two approved medications in this class, to help control rising glucose levels after meals. These medications, however, aren't appropriate for anyone with gastroparesis.

Synthetic amylin, or Symlin. Just arriving on the market after almost two decades of research is a new medication, Symlin (generic name pramlintide), a synthetic form of a natural hormone (**amylin**) normally coreleased with insulin by your pancreatic beta cells. If your body makes very little or none of its own insulin, then you are missing the natural release of this hormone. Symlin is the first new treatment for people with type 1 diabetes in over eight decades (since the discovery of insulin in 1921); however, it has been approved for use in people with type 2 diabetes who also take insulin.

One drawback of its use is that this synthetic form of amylin must be injected like insulin. Its main action is to work with insulin following meals to control the flow of glucose into your circulation coming from the food that you ate. The main side effects of Symlin are the potential for severe hypoglycemia (the risk is greater in type 1 users), nausea, vomiting, abdominal pain, headache, fatigue, and dizziness. People with gastroparesis should not use this medication as it can cause them to develop more frequent severe hypoglycemia. A potential additional benefit is that Symlin can help you lose some weight, possibly due to tighter BG control and early satiety; a further benefit is that it may reduce oxidative stress and prevent you from developing diabetic complications.

Incretins and incretin mimetics. Finally, a new class of diabetic medications known as **incretins** or incretin mimetics has recently been approved for use in the treatment of type 2 diabetes. These compounds, which are actually synthetic versions of a small protein derived from the venom of the Gila monster (a poisonous lizard found in the southwestern United States and Mexico), appear to simultaneously stimulate the initial release of insulin in response to any food you eat (a response that is missing in most people with diabetes); protect your pancreatic beta cells from burnout (the main reason for the failure of other diabetic drugs such as sulfonylureas); inhibit your liver's release of glucose (by blocking glucagon release); delay the emptying of food from your stomach; and promote early feelings of fullness—usually causing you to lose weight.

One of these compounds (exenatide, a compound that agonizes incretin receptors) recently received FDA approval under the trade name Byetta. Despite occasional side effects such as nausea, vomiting, transient headaches, and increased risk of hypoglycemia when used with sulfonylureas, this newest class of medications effectively replaces natural hormones normally released by the digestive tract after meals to spur insulin release and provides another choice for diabetes treatment, particularly if your treatment with sulfonylureas or other compounds is no longer working effectively. A drawback for many potential users, though, is that it has to be injected (rather than ingested) twice a day.

Combination therapies. It's much better for your health if you can avoid having extended periods of hyperglycemia, so if you can't adequately control your BG levels within the first three to six months on a medication like a biguanide (metformin) despite increasing dosages, your physician should talk to you about adding additional therapies. Due to the progressive nature of diabetes, even if your physician put you on only one diabetic medication to start, it's not uncommon to end up being prescribed two or more to use simultaneously. In fact, the standard medical practice when the first prescribed medication fails to adequately control your BG levels is to add in another—thus initiating a **combination therapy**—without stopping the first one.

Other medications that you can potentially supplement with include sulfonylureas (e.g., Glynase or Glucotrol), which work by stimulating your pancreas to produce more insulin. Originally the only prescribed medication available to treat type 2 diabetes, the newer generation of medications in this class have fewer potential side effects than the older ones. Nevertheless, they are of limited use since your pancreas may eventually lose the capacity to make much insulin, at which point no medication is going to be able to stimulate your beta cells to make enough to control your BG levels effectively. Unfortunately, a new study recently showed that although your glycemic control may initially be improved by adding a sulfonylurea to a biguanide, your BG levels are likely to resume their deterioration in as little as six months after you start using both medications together. Fortunately, though, newer compounds such as Byetta have recently been shown to be extremely effective in reversing this downward spiral and lowering your BG levels once maximal doses of combination oral therapies have begun to fail.

The future of oral medications. New diabetes-related medications are coming on the market at a rapid rate, and it's hard at this point to know exactly what the future holds for diabetes treatment. Just two decades ago, the only oral medications available to treat diabetes were the sulfonylureas, which are now woefully inadequate in most cases at controlling BG levels on their own. Combination therapies are currently at the forefront of diabetes management, but new advances will change the course of future treatment. In addition, recently discovered genes that may be responsible for weight gain and type 2 diabetes may be the new targets of the next generation of medications; diabetes may even be prevented in the first place. Finally, immune suppression alone or in combination with therapies promoting beta cell regrowth may enable your own pancreas to start producing adequate amounts of insulin again.

TIP

37

NO MATTER YOUR WEIGHT

SOME PHYSICIANS feel that weight-reducing drugs may play a more prominent role in the prevention and treatment of type 2 diabetes in the coming years. In the meantime, use a more natural approach of positive lifestyle changes to achieve similar results.

Insulin use

Being put on insulin is not a sign that you have somehow personally failed at controlling your diabetes, which is your primary goal. Regardless of the type, diabetes results in a progressive loss of your beta cells and a lessening of your insulin-producing capacity over time. Consequently, all people with type 1 diabetes and at least 40 percent of people who have type 2 ultimately have to use supplemental injections of insulin to even come close to adequately controlling their BG levels. If your BG level is quite high when you are diagnosed (greater than 250 mg/dl), your physician may choose to initiate medications including insulin immediately; this may later be decreased or withdrawn if your lifestyle changes are effective at controlling your diabetes. When you're newly diagnosed with type 2, starting on insulin immediately can allow you to rapidly achieve good control. In fact, doing so may have a positive residual effect, because when people with type 2 diabetes are started on insulin early, they are not likely to still need supplemental insulin a year later.

Long-acting insulins. If or when you have to start using insulin for better control, you have a choice of a number of different insulin regimens. For starters, you can use insulin in combination with other medications, such as Precose or Glyset, taken with meals to slow down carbohydrate absorption. You can also use once- or twice-a-day dosing with some of the **long-acting insulin** choices, which provide basal insulin coverage to give your body the extra insulin it needs without food intake. These include Lantus (insulin glargine, the first long-acting basal insulin **analog**, which covers basal insulin needs for 24 hours) and Levemir (an alternate basal analog known generically as insulin detemir, recently approved by the FDA).

The main difference between these two long-acting synthetic insulins (altered slightly for more even absorption over time) is that Levemir is being marketed for use once *or* twice daily (although most people would need twice-daily injections) with supposedly more even absorption and insulin coverage than Lantus, which is marketed for once-a-day use. In my experience with Lantus, if you take small doses of 10 or fewer units per injection, it may not last a full 24 hours, and most people (especially those with type 1 diabetes) will need to dose with it twice daily. An older long-acting insulin, Ultralente (U), was just taken out of production permanently. Prior to the introduction of Lantus, U was the long-acting insulin of choice, but it fell out of favor with many insulin users because of its longer duration (48 hours) and definite peak. These two newer analogs are virtually peakless, meaning that the insulin is provided in almost even amounts over their duration.

Intermediate-acting insulin. Another choice of many physicians is NPH (N), an intermediate-acting insulin. Some practitioners prescribe oral medications during the day and an injection at bedtime to prevent your fasting BG from being too elevated in the morning. Unfortunately, if you use any insulin, you're likely to gain some weight, but combining daytime oral medications with evening injections of N appears to minimize that weight gain. Although the manufacturers of Levemir claim that it does not cause its users to gain weight, that claim has yet to be proven; Lantus itself causes some weight gain, but less than a 70/30 mixture of NovoLog (30 percent), a rapid-acting insulin, and a slower-release form of it (70 percent) that acts similarly to N. Another combination option that has been used successfully once glycemia is under better control with insulin is to add in Glucophage and then lower or stop using the insulin.

The Action of Insulin and Insulin Analogs

INSULIN	ONSET	PEAK	DURATION
Humalog/NovoLog/Apidra	10–30 minutes	0.5–3 hours	3–5 hours
Regular (R)	30–60 minutes	2–5 hours	5–8 hours
NPH (N)/Lente (L)	1–2 hours	2–12 hours	14–24 hours
Lantus	1.5 hours	None	20–24 hours
Levemir	1–3 hours	8–10 hours	Up to 24 hours

Rapid-acting insulin analogs. If you aren't able to control your BG levels with any of the longer-acting insulins alone, **rapid-acting insulin analogs**, such as Humalog, NovoLog, and Apidra, all of which exert their main effects within thirty minutes to three hours after a bolus injection, can also be prescribed for you to dose with during meals and snacks. Insulin analogs have become extremely popular since their introduction to the market over a decade ago (starting with Humalog, then NovoLog, and recently Apidra). An insulin analog is a slightly altered form of human insulin that has undergone substitution of a different amino acid or two somewhere in the normal insulin protein chain, which causes it to be absorbed more rapidly (or more evenly, in the case of the basal analogs) from skin injection sites than normal insulin. All of these analogs have a fairly similar onset of action, peak, and duration. In research studies, Humalog and NovoLog cause similar improvements in your BG control; Apidra (insulin glulisine), however, just recently gained FDA approval and has not been as fully researched as the first two. You can also use regular (R) insulin (synthetic human insulin, not an insulin analog) similarly for food intake, but it is considered "short-acting" rather than "rapid" as it has a slower onset and longer duration than the newer synthetic analogs.

TIP

38

NO MATTER YOUR WEIGHT

IF YOU take oral diabetic medications or use insulin regimens, they can cause you to gain weight. To avoid this weight gain, aim to be able to lower the doses of all your diabetes medications with regular physical activity and a low-GI diet. You may also choose to use the medications that usually cause weight loss, including Glucophage (not the XR form, though), Symlin (if you use insulin), or Byetta.

Insulin pumps. Whether you have type 1 or type 2 diabetes, if you use insulin, you may choose to use an insulin pump, which is a subcutaneous catheter device programmed to continuously deliver small, basal doses of short-acting insulin (to mimic the coverage of the longer-acting options), along with bolus doses of the same to cover your carbohydrate intake at meals and snacks. Many models of insulin pumps are now available, and the features vary by manufacturer and model; to find the one that is right for you, talk with your health-care provider. You can also research and compare the various models on your own either by looking online at the Diabetes Mall (www.diabetesnet.com) or obtaining a copy of the annual spring issue of *Diabetes Health* magazine (www.DiabetesHealth.com), which provides an extremely comprehensive product reference and comparison guide.

Inhaled insulins. If you dislike needles and have been avoiding using insulin for that reason, take heart; it appears that alternate insulin delivery methods are on the not-so-distant horizon. While trials of inhaled insulins such as Exubera (coproduced by Pfizer and Aventis) have resulted in some negative effects on the lung function of some of its experimental users, it's still expected to hit the market by 2006, with competitors' versions of inhaled insulin appearing shortly thereafter. A recent trial demonstrated that inhaled insulin may actually hit your bloodstream faster than any injected type, making it ideal for controlling your after-meal BG spikes and perhaps eliminating your need for basal insulin injections (which inhaled insulin wouldn't be able to replace anyway), as long as your body still makes some of its own insulin. In addition, recent clinical trials on short-acting forms of **oral insulin** (Oralin) have been extremely promising. When delivered into your mouth in a fine spray in measured doses before meals, it is rapidly absorbed and capable of controlling your BG levels at least as effectively as equivalent doses of injected premeal insulin. At this time, though, it is not considered an effective replacement for basal insulin therapies, such as Lantus, Levemir, or insulin pumps.

Exercise precautions when using oral diabetic medications

Certain medications, including some of the oral diabetic medications, can affect your body's response to exercise. These medications, as I discussed previously, target one or more of the metabolic dysfunctions a diabetic state creates: insulin release from the pancreatic beta cells, the liver's production of BG, and insulin resistance in fat tissues, the liver, or muscles. Depending on their path of action, they may or may not affect your glycemic responses to physical activity.

Certain sulfonylureas increase your risk of developing hypoglycemia. Older-generation sulfonylureas (such as Diabinese and Orinase) cause insulin release from the pancreas and somewhat decrease insulin resistance. However, these older medications typically have a longer duration (up to 72 hours) and, therefore, have the greatest potential to cause a low BG level during and/or following exercise. Second-generation sulfonylureas, such as Amaryl, DiaBeta, Micronase, and Glucotrol, generally don't last as long and carry a smaller risk; of these, DiaBeta and Micronase carry the greatest risk due to their slightly longer duration (24 hours versus only 12 to 16 hours for the others). You will have to frequently monitor your BG levels when exercising if you take any of the listed sulfonylureas that stay in your system longer; and, when your exercise becomes regular enough, you may need to check with your health-care provider about lowering your doses of these medications if you are frequently experiencing hypoglycemia during or following exercise.

Other medications may have less of an effect on exercise. Insulin sensitizers like Avandia and Actos mainly affect the action of your insulin at rest, not during exercise, so the risk of these medications causing exercise hypoglycemia is almost nonexistent. Similarly, Glucophage is unlikely to cause exercise lows. Prandin or Starlix would only potentially increase your risk of a low BG level if taken immediately before prolonged exercise, since they increase insulin levels in the blood only temporarily when taken with meals. Finally, medications that slow down the absorption of carbohydrates (Precose and Glyset) would not directly affect exercise, but could slightly delay your treatment of a low BG level since you would have to take in carbohydrates to treat it, and thus their absorption would be slowed.

Insulin and exercise interactions

If you use supplemental insulin, you face a potentially more complicated exercise-medication interaction. Understanding the effects of insulin action and different regimens on glycemic control is one of the best strategies for optimizing exercise management. As I discussed previously, insulin and muscular contractions evoke separate mechanisms that cause you to take up glucose into your muscles, and they additively increase muscle glucose uptake; thus, the type of insulin that you use and the timing of its use can have a large effect on glycemic responses. You may be one of the many individuals who use a combination of short- and long-acting insulins (varying by time to peak action and total duration) given two to four (or more) times daily. Or you may receive a continuous infusion of short-acting insulin through an insulin pump.

When no more than basal levels of insulin are circulating in your body during exercise, your physiological response will be more normal, more like someone who doesn't have diabetes. If you exercise when your insulin levels are peaking, however, you'll have an increased risk of hypoglycemia. For example, if you inject intermediate-acting N at breakfast, it will peak around noon and exert its effects throughout the afternoon; if you exercise then, your BG level may drop more rapidly than at other times. In contrast, Lantus provides only basal insulin coverage for 24 hours, making a separate dose of short-acting insulin required to cover lunch if your body no longer makes much insulin. Thus, if you use Lantus either by itself, with no rapid-acting insulin, or your last injection of rapid-acting insulin has peaked and waned before you start exercising, your risk of a low BG level will be much lower. Similarly, insulin pump users can normalize their response to exercise by either disconnecting their pumps or reducing programmed basal rates during physical activity; some users also decrease their basal rates before and/or after the activity, depending on how long it lasts and on their individual BG responses.

Exercise effects of changes in insulin action

A multitude of other variables affecting insulin action can confound your glycemic responses to exercise. For example, if you exercise in the morning before taking any insulin, the result is usually a lesser decline in your BG level compared with the same exercise done later in the day; this is due to elevations in cortisol and growth hormone you experience in the morning after an overnight fast, which serve to increase insulin resistance. Thus, you will generally need to make fewer changes to your food intake or medications for morning exercise. Exercising in the late evening, though, sets you up with the biggest risk of postexercise hypoglycemia, especially overnight during sleep, but you can still do it safely if you take certain precautions, such as eating a bedtime snack or lowering your bedtime insulin dose (particularly if you take N insulin in the evening or at bedtime).

If you're physically fit, you generally have a heightened sensitivity to insulin, allowing glucose to enter your muscle cells more efficiently both during exercise and while you rest. The short-term increase in your glucose uptake likely results from greater rates of muscle glycogen repletion right after exercise. However, at least one research study showed that, following a competitive marathon completed with normal BG levels, type 1 participants had unchanged insulin sensitivity the following morning despite having used significant amounts of their glycogen depletion the previous day. They were likely experiencing an increased fat use after such exhaustive exercise, which is normal even for people without diabetes, and they likely had some micro damage to their muscles that was keeping them from rapidly replacing their muscle glycogen. Any longer-term changes in your insulin sensitivity, however, are more reflective of adaptive changes in your muscle tissue from training that increase your BG uptake into cells by insulin-sensitive glucose transport proteins. These changes will usually cause your total insulin needs to drop, regardless of which insulin regimen you follow, and you may have to adjust your insulin doses downward to compensate. You must exercise regularly, though, as this heightened insulin sensitivity begins to decline after a day or two of inactivity, which is why becoming a regular exerciser is crucial to optimizing your BG control.

Do you need to worry about other medications and exercise?

Besides taking medications for BG control, you—like many people with diabetes—may also need help controlling your blood lipids (especially cholesterol levels), hypertension, and other coexisting health problems. Most medications taken for nondiabetic reasons will not affect your exercise response directly—with a few notable exceptions. **Medications with potential effects on exercise.** Certain medications taken to treat high cholesterol levels or abnormal levels of blood fats common in diabetes (i.e., the "**statins**," including Lipitor, Mevacor, Pravachol, Crestor, and Zocor) may result in unexplained muscle pain and weakness with physical activity, possibly by compromising your muscles' ability to generate energy; however, case reports of muscle cramps during or after exercise, nocturnal cramping, and general fatigue show that these symptoms resolve when you discontinue taking the statins. If you are taking a statin and experience any of these symptoms, talk with your doctor about possibly switching to another type of cholesterol-lowering drug. Furthermore, any medications taken to reduce your body water levels (diuretics like Lasix, Microzide, Enduron, and Lozol) and improve your blood pressure can lead to dehydration and dizziness from hypotension (low blood pressure) more easily, but will not likely affect your BG levels, although they may interfere with your body's secretion of insulin. Vasodilators such as nitroglycerin allow more blood to flow to your heart during exercise, but they can also induce hypotension, which may cause you to faint during or following an activity. You'll also experience a dramatic effect with beta-blockers (Lopressor, Inderal, Levatol, Corgard, Tenormin, Zebeta, and others) taken to treat heart disease and hypertension, as they lower both your resting and exercise heart rates; if you are taking a blocker, your heart rate will not reach any age-expected value at any intensity of exercise.

Medications with no exercise effects. You may also be taking either **ACE inhibitors** (Capoten, Accupril, Vasotec, Lotensin, Zestril, etc.) or **angiotensin II receptor blockers** (ARBs, such as Cozaar, Benicar, and Avapro) to reduce your blood pressure and/or protect your kidneys from possible damage. If you take either of these types of medications, you should expect no negative effects during exercise. In fact, using certain ACE inhibitors may *lower* your risk of untoward cardiovascular events if you have heart disease. Other medications taken to treat heart disease and hypertension (calcium-channel blockers like Procardia, Sular, Cardene, Cardizem, and Norvasc), depression (Wellbutrin, Prozac, and others), or chronic pain (Celebrex) will have no effect on your ability to exercise safely and effectively. However, keep in mind that aspirin and other blood thinners (such as Coumadin) have the potential to make you bruise more easily or extensively in response to athletic injuries.

Are nutritional supplements right for you?

The need for supplemental vitamins, minerals, and other compounds may still be hotly debated in the nutritional world, but the reality is that consumers like you and me already spend billions of dollars a year on them. While some experts claim that you can get everything your body needs by simply consuming a nutritionally balanced diet, many others loudly denounce these claims, asserting that nutritional supplements are absolutely necessary, especially if you have a chronic health condition like diabetes. The evidence suggests that diabetes itself creates a special metabolic situation—particularly when your BG is not well controlled—that may raise your risk for depletion of certain nutrients, which you may be able to offset by adding in healthier food choices and/or nutritional supplements.

Before self-prescribing any supplements, though, try to assess your true need for them. If you are taking in the recommended daily amounts of vitamins and minerals, then you might not need supplements. For them to be effective, you usually must be deficient in whichever nutrients they are providing. While insulin resistance and hyperglycemia can potentially cause certain nutrient deficiencies, if you control these conditions with the seven steps outlined in this book, then supplements may not be of any additional help.

TIP

39

NO MATTER YOUR WEIGHT

DON'T BELIEVE everything you read when it comes to health claims about nutritional supplements, as the scientific evidence is often conflicting and inconclusive. For example, recent studies reported that conjugated linoleic acid (CLA)—widely used as a weight-loss supplement—may actually increase insulin resistance in obese men, while others touted its supposed role in *preventing* insulin resistance–associated cardiovascular disease in people with diabetes. The jury is still out on what its effects may be if you have both excess body weight and diabetes.

Try a combination nutritional supplement

If you decide that you need to take supplements, a combination may be most effective. One combination that improves levels of the "good" cholesterol in people with diabetes (at least in one study) is vitamins C and E and minerals magnesium and zinc. No one combination may work for everyone, so if you do decide to supplement, do it scientifically: have your glycated hemoglobin and lipid levels tested before you start supplementing, and then again no sooner than three months later. If you see improvements and you haven't changed anything else (such as your diet or exercise regimens), then the supplements may be benefiting you. Unfortunately, if you take supplements purely for their antioxidant properties, there is no easy way to assess whether they are having the hoped-for impact.

As for other supplements, a lot of myths are circulating about their health benefits, and in many cases, no definitive answers have been reached even through well-grounded, scientific research. For instance, a recent study concluded that green tea may improve insulin sensitivity and lower blood pressure—at least in fructose-fed rats that had large doses of powdered green tea dissolved in their drinking water. Regrettably, this effect is as yet unproven in humans, and even if it were, we're unlikely to consume green tea in equivalent amounts to these rats given our much more significant body weights.

Finding the Nutrient Content of Supplements

THE METABOLIC effects of most nutrients are frequently synergistic with others found in whole foods in their natural state, which you aren't likely to get when you ingest a particular nutrient in supplement form. For more information on the nutrient content of supplements and foods, access any of several government Web sites, including www.nal.usda.gov/fnic/foodcomp, www.cc.nih.gov/ccc/supplements, and/or www.cfsan.fda.gov/~dms/supplmnt.html.

The power of antioxidants. Oxygen free radicals that can damage cells are produced and then quenched by antioxidant enzyme systems in your body all the time—in fact, they are even created by exercise. Regular physical activity, though, increases the power of the antioxidant energy systems that you have in your body. The problem arises when more oxidative stress occurs than your body can handle, and elevated BG is one of the conditions that can trigger oxidative damage caused by excess free radicals. The accumulation of oxidative stress due to hyperglycemia may ultimately contribute to the development of most of the complications associated with long-term diabetes, including heart disease and eye, kidney, and nerve damage. High levels of BG, elevated circulating insulin, and insulin resistance together enhance free radical production if you have diabetes, and these radical compounds then promote further insulin resistance and a lower insulin secretion, thereby creating a downhill spiral for insulin action in your body.

Diabetes and antioxidant nutrients. Among the most popular diabetes-related supplements are a variety of antioxidant vitamins and minerals. Normally, your body possesses enough antioxidant enzymes to be able to fight most or all of the free radicals that are created. Diabetes, however, packs a double punch to these enzymes: not only is free-radical generation increased by hyperglycemia, but it also depresses your body's natural antioxidant defenses. Thus, if your BG levels are poorly controlled, you are among the most likely to benefit from supplemental antioxidant therapies. While certain oral diabetic medications (e.g., gliclazide, a sulfonylurea used outside of the United States) can potentially lower oxidative stress, antioxidant nutrients are the most effective way to complement or augment your body's own ability to combat the abundance of these compounds when you have diabetes.

Specific dietary antioxidants appear to be of particular benefit in treating and preventing diabetes and its complications, including vitamin E, vitamin C, beta-carotene, **glutathione, alpha lipoic acid**, selenium, copper, and zinc. CoQ_{10}, also known as coenzyme Q and ubiquinone, may also have an antioxidant role, but hasn't been as widely studied to date. Antioxidants are believed to be integrally involved in the prevention of many diabetic complications, such as cataracts, which result at least partially from deficient glutathione levels leading to a faulty antioxidant defense system within the lens of your eye. Nutrients such as lipoic acid, vitamins E and C, and selenium can increase your levels of glutathione and its activity, allowing for better protection of your eyes and other tissues. Taking too much of these disease-fighting compounds in the form of large supplemental doses can be counterproductive, though, as almost all antioxidants have been shown to have the opposite effect when taken in unnaturally large doses.

Antioxidants naturally in foods. It's impossible to overdose on antioxidants if you obtain them naturally through food, so it's far better to consume them that way whenever possible. Some surprising foods and drinks contain large amounts of various antioxidants. For example, a recent study found that a typical cup of hot cocoa (containing two tablespoons of pure cocoa powder) has twice as many of these health-promoting compounds (flavonoids in particular) as red wine, two to three times more than green tea, and almost five times more than black tea. Drinking cocoa hot also apparently releases more antioxidant power (but remember to use the sugar-free variety for better diabetes control).

Vitamin E. Vitamin E, comprising a family of tocopherols that scavenges peroxyl radicals that damage cell membranes around your body, is one of only four fat-soluble vitamins. As such, it's able to effectively prevent the oxidation of unsaturated (good) fats in various membranes around the body, including those found in red blood cells, nerves, and lungs. This vitamin also reduces oxidative stress in your arteries, which can reduce plaque formation there, in part by making LDL cholesterol less susceptible to oxidation and impairing its ability to accelerate heart disease.

Unfortunately, recent research has suggested that vitamin E supplements may not only be ineffective at combating cardiovascular disease, but in some cases may also contribute to the development of heart failure. Moreover, combining its intake with Lipitor (a cholesterol-lowering drug taken by many people with type 2 diabetes) may also have detrimental effects. The supplements, most of which contain only the dl-alpha tocopherol form of this vitamin, are not as effective as having all forms of tocopherol compounds (alpha, delta, gamma, and others) together, which you can only get naturally in foods. A few more expensive supplements contain at least several forms of these tocopherols, but research has not yet tested their effectiveness in combating oxidative stress, so it's too early to say whether they're worth the extra money.

Nevertheless, vitamin E supplements of any kind may be effective in combating excessive oxidation of other fats, a major cause of diabetes-related tissue damage in your eyes (cataract formation), nerves (tingling, numbness, and pain), muscles (weakness and atrophy), and immune cells (increased susceptibility to infections). Furthermore, low serum levels of vitamin E have been associated with a greater risk of developing type 2 diabetes, so it is certainly good to eat more foods that contain it. This vitamin can be found naturally in vegetable oils, seeds (especially sunflower seeds), nuts (particularly almonds), green, leafy vegetables (such as spinach and broccoli), margarine, fortified breakfast cereals, tomato products, sweet potatoes, and wheat germ. Unfortunately, cooking and food processing may destroy it, making it difficult for you to consume adequate amounts.

Vitamin E supplements can be taken to correct any deficiencies, but keep in mind that unless you read the label to find the ones with several tocopherols, your supplement is only likely to contain the alpha form of this vitamin, which means that it may not be very effective. You can take up to 800 international units (IU) safely as a daily supplement.

Vitamin C. Ascorbic acid, otherwise known as vitamin C, is a water-soluble vitamin with strong antioxidant qualities. Think about what happens to a sliced apple when it sits out on the counter: the exposed inner surfaces start to turn brown due to the oxygen in the air. You can prevent this oxidation by coating the apple with lemon or orange juice, both of which are high in vitamin C.

While deficiencies of this vitamin are rare in the United States, lower blood levels of vitamin C have been found in those who are insulin resistant and at high risk for developing type 2 diabetes. Although this vitamin is generally considered to be less effective in combating diabetic complications than vitamin E or other antioxidants, if you use it as a supplement, it should reduce your blood pressure and improve the elasticity of your arterial walls—both of which reduce your risk of heart disease. It also plays a definite role in the prevention and treatment of diabetic eye diseases, including cataracts and glaucoma (the second leading cause of new blindness), likely because oxidative stress is a major factor in their development.

Vitamin C is abundant in more than just citrus fruits. You can also find it in bell peppers, peaches, strawberries, broccoli, and salad greens, and it is added to many other foods as a preservative (just look for "ascorbate" on the ingredients list). Thus, the recommended intake of 200 mg per day can easily be obtained through food intake. Taking megadoses of supplemental vitamin C is still controversial; doses of 1,000 milligrams per day or more may contribute to the formation of kidney stones or result in rebound scurvy (a disease affecting collagen that vitamin C normally prevents) when you stop taking large supplements of it. Another recent study, on postmenopausal women with type 2 diabetes, found an association between large vitamin C supplements and increased risk of dying from heart disease. Given these potential risks, vitamin C is best obtained naturally through your diet or through smaller doses of no more than 200 milligrams per day.

Beta-carotene and vitamin A. Beta-carotene, one compound in a family of carotenoids, may not be a first-line antioxidant in the body, but it does boost the activity of your tumor-scavenging, natural killer cells, which are an integral part of your cell-based immune system. Along with other antioxidants, it also helps inhibit cholesterol synthesis, facilitate cellular interactions, and stimulate enzymes to repair damaged DNA. This provitamin by itself is not active without being converted by your body into **retinol**, the active form of vitamin A. Retinol is involved in maintaining the health of the retina (the back of the eye, which is often damaged by diabetes), immune system, skin, epithelial cells (which line the organs and are where cancers start), and memory.

It makes no difference if you consume beta-carotene instead of vitamin A, as your body will convert it into the active form as needed. It's better to focus on beta-carotene intake, which can be accomplished by eating yellow-orange vegetables such as carrots, pumpkin, squash, and sweet potatoes; green, leafy vegetables such as spinach, kale, turnip greens, and broccoli; tomato products; and fruits such as cantaloupe, oranges, limes, pineapple, and prunes. A glass of milk provides about 15 percent of your recommended daily intake, while a medium carrot supplies much more, at 200 percent. Taking supplements of beta-carotene is generally less effective than consuming this provitamin in its natural form, not least as foods also contain other carotenoids, including alpha-carotene, that are currently proving to be even more effective cancer fighters than the beta form.

Megadoses of beta-carotene are generally considered to be harmless, but you really shouldn't need supplements, since a balanced diet supplies more than adequate amounts of beta-carotene. Vitamin A, on the other hand, is toxic if you take it in large doses, which you can only do through dietary supplements. Retinol is found mainly in foods such as liver, butter, cheese, egg yolks, fish liver oils, and fortified milk; in fact, a single serving of liver provides 1,000 percent of the recommended dietary intake. The upper limit for daily intake of vitamin A is 10,000 IU; beta-carotene has no limit.

Glutathione and alpha lipoic acid. Glutathione is the main antioxidant enzyme found in all of your cells. This substance, along with alpha lipoic acid (ALA), is the most important antioxidant in your body. Composed of three amino acids found abundantly in foods, glutathione protects the DNA in your cell nuclei from being oxidized. Your body can produce both glutathione and ALA, but may not always synthesize enough to meet your needs, especially when these needs are elevated by diabetes. It can also be obtained naturally from various vegetables and fruits, such as asparagus, avocados, spinach, strawberries, peaches, melons, and citrus fruits.

While ALA increases glutathione levels by helping cells absorb a critical amino acid needed for its synthesis, it also guards against common diabetic complications, including stroke, heart attacks, peripheral nerve damage, and cataracts, as well as memory loss, cancer, and aging effects. Spinach (raw or cooked) is the best source of this nutrient, also found naturally in small amounts in broccoli, tomatoes, potatoes, peas, and Brussels sprouts. Spinach is especially touted for its ability to fight diabetic cataracts and macular degeneration (the leading cause of blindness in all adults) rather than for its iron content.

If you have diabetes, these two natural antioxidants may be even more vital. Glutathione levels are depleted by elevated BG levels in various tissues around the body, leaving the door wide open for increased oxidative damage when your diabetes is not well controlled. In fact, it is of utmost importance to maintain normal levels of glutathione to prevent diabetic cataracts. As for ALA, it has been shown to have the ability to normalize diabetes-induced kidney dysfunction and to lower other biomarkers of oxidative stress, including potential damage to your nerve cells, where it additionally promotes nerve fiber regeneration and stimulates a substance known as nerve growth factor. So, now's the time to start eating spinach at least a couple of times a week.

Selenium. This **trace mineral** is essential for the proper functioning of numerous enzymes in your body, particularly one of the body's antioxidant enzymes, glutathione peroxidase, which works along with vitamin E to prevent damage to the membranes of your oxygen-carrying red blood cells (among others). While this mineral does not have the capacity to lower BG levels, it is believed to play an important role in the prevention of diabetic cataracts, as well as cardiovascular disease (by preventing oxidation of LDL cholesterol), and even prostate, colon, and lung cancers. In a recent study pooling data on more than seventeen hundred people, those with higher blood levels of selenium had a 34 percent lower risk of colon cancer than those with lower levels.

Brazil nuts are a particularly good source of selenium (one nut contains a full day's supply), but you can also obtain it by eating adequate amounts of most seafood; organ meats such as liver; poultry; and whole-grain products grown in selenium-rich soil (found in most parts of the United States). The recommended daily intake of selenium is currently 55 micrograms (mcg). If you take it as a supplement, your dose should not exceed 200 mcg daily, or it may impair the synthesis of thyroid hormones that elevate your metabolism.

Copper. This trace mineral is a component (along with zinc) of another antioxidant enzyme in your body called superoxide dismutase (SOD). Copper deficiency due to inadequate dietary intake is not known to exist in humans, but your copper levels may be lower if you have diabetes. Decreased levels of SOD have been found in diabetic people with kidney disease, along with markers of increased oxidative stress and inflammation. Elevated levels of SOD, on the other hand, have prevented the destruction of pancreatic beta cells in studies of animals with type 1 diabetes. In addition, it works in concert with iron to help form hemoglobin, the compound that binds and carries oxygen in your blood for delivery to cells around your body.

This nutrient can be found in beef, shellfish, whole-grain products, baking chocolate, mushrooms, nuts (cashews, Brazil nuts, walnuts), sunflower seeds, legumes, potatoes, avocados, broccoli, bananas, and couscous. The recommended daily intake is 0.9 mg, with an upper limit of 10 mg. Supplements are not recommended, as taking in excessive copper can cause nausea and vomiting, as well as copper poisoning.

Zinc. Another trace mineral, zinc is a component of more than one hundred enzymes, many of which are involved in glucose metabolism. A mild dietary zinc deficiency is thought to be common in the United States, particularly if your intake of animal protein is relatively low. It's mainly found in oysters and other shellfish, meats, and poultry, although lesser amounts are available in whole grains, dairy products, fortified breakfast cereals, semisweet chocolate, nuts, and seeds. Zinc lozenges are also widely available in drug and food stores as a way to alleviate the common cold (although this role has not been conclusively proven).

Having diabetes apparently affects your zinc status, potentially resulting in a deficiency as you lose more of it through your urine when your BG level is high. Since zinc plays a clear role in the synthesis, storage, and secretion of insulin from functional beta cells, a deficiency may interfere with your normal release of insulin if you have type 2 diabetes. Furthermore, some diabetic complications, such as changes to the retina in the eye, may be related to increased oxidative stress associated with decreases in zinc, as the function of the SOD enzyme (mentioned in relation to copper) is also dependent on the availability of adequate zinc.

Some practitioners may make a case for zinc supplements if you are truly deficient. However, be forewarned that supplements containing even 25 mg per day (the recommended intake is 8 to 11 mg for adults) may interfere with the absorption of other minerals, such as copper and iron, even though the upper intake level for zinc via supplements is currently set at 40 mg daily. Doses of over 100 mg daily may actually increase the "bad" cholesterol in your blood while decreasing the "good" type, as well as contribute to the development of anemia. Therefore, only a low-dose supplement would be advisable, and only if you can't take in adequate zinc through your diet alone.

The antidiabetic effect of certain vitamins and supplements

Vitamin D. Another fat-soluble vitamin best known for its hormone-like role in increasing your body's absorption of dietary calcium, vitamin D promotes bone health and likely also muscle strength. Diabetes causes bone-mineral loss, particularly from the long bones in your legs and arms, regardless of how successful you are with diabetes control. In addition to adequate intake of vitamin D, bone health is known to require sufficient intake of vitamin K, calcium, magnesium, and zinc. Interestingly, the role that vitamin B_{12} may additionally play in bone health was just recently assessed, and it appears that low blood levels of this B vitamin are linked to lower bone density in the spines of women and the hips of men. Folic acid (also known as folate) is another B vitamin that is currently being studied for its potential role in promoting stronger bones, so make sure that you are getting the daily recommended intake of these two vitamins (6 mcg for vitamin B_{12} and 400 mcg for folic acid). As an added bonus, folate will likely reduce your chances of developing cardiovascular disease or having a stroke.

A vitamin D deficiency may have a much greater negative impact on people with diabetes than was originally suspected, partly contributing to impairments in your insulin secretion and action—particularly during the winter when your vitamin D levels may be low. The biologically active form of vitamin D is a potent modulator of your immune system, and a deficiency may contribute to the development of autoimmune-based type 1 diabetes. Moreover, emerging evidence suggests that low vitamin D status is even a risk factor for type 2 diabetes and prediabetes, as a deficiency of this vitamin appears to worsen pancreatic beta cell function. Unfortunately, though, most foods do not naturally contain any of this vitamin, so it's difficult to get enough of it through your diet. It can be obtained through fortified dairy products, margarine, and fish oils; one glass of vitamin D–fortified milk or soy milk will provide 25 percent of currently recommended daily requirements.

But the best way to get enough of this vitamin is through exposure to sunlight, during which the UV-B rays convert vitamin D_3, a prohormone, into **calcitriol**, the active form of this vitamin. In order for this conversion to take place, you must expose at least your hands, arms, and face to sunlight two to three times per week. Those with lighter-colored skin can get the UV exposure they need in about 10 to 15 minutes, but darker-skinned people have to spend up to a couple of hours in the sun to make enough vitamin D. Longer exposure is also needed during the winter, and so your vitamin D may be deficient during the winter months, especially if you live in northern latitudes where UV-B rays are not sufficient many months during the year.

Concern over skin cancer has led more people to wear UV-ray sunscreen, which largely inhibits production of vitamin D. Just recently, though, some dermatologists have begun to reconsider the current guidelines for use of sunscreen products and to recommend a lesser use of them. The risk of dying from skin cancer is low, and emerging evidence suggests that higher vitamin D levels actually protect you against the development of skin melanomas. In other words, if you block too much of the sun's rays, you may actually be increasing your risk of skin (and other, deadlier) cancers rather than preventing them.

Also unfortunate is the fact that the skin's ability to make vitamin D via sun exposure declines significantly with age, which means that few older adults actually reach the recommended daily levels of vitamin D intake. For this reason, the National Academy of Sciences has set the latest vitamin D daily intake recommendations on an age-related scale: 200 IU—about the amount found in two eight-ounce glasses of milk—for those 19 to 50 years of age; 400 IU for those aged 51 to 70 years; and 600 IU for people 70 and older. A growing number of scientists, however, believe that vitamin D intake should be at least 1,000 IU or higher, regardless of your age. At this time, the tolerable upper intake is 2,000 IU for all adults, and toxic levels have been reported at 10,000 IU or higher per day. Any supplements that you take should contain vitamin D_3 rather than the less active form (ergocalciferol, or vitamin D_2).

Cinnamon. At least one spice has been touted for its potential antidiabetic effects: cinnamon. It appears to contain bioactive phenols (chemical compounds) that act as phytonutrients. While the scientific studies on its effects in humans are few, at least one study has shown that intake of 1, 3, or 6 grams of cinnamon per day reduces your BG, triglycerides (circulating blood fats), LDL, and total cholesterol if you have type 2 diabetes.

Minerals with antidiabetic effects

Magnesium. The fourth most abundant mineral in the body, magnesium is widely distributed in foods, particularly in seafood, nuts (Brazil nuts, almonds, and cashews, for example), green leafy vegetables (e.g., spinach), other fruits and vegetables (including bananas), whole-grain products, oat bran, semisweet chocolate, and legumes. Magnesium is an integral component of more than three hundred enzymes, most of which affect your muscles' metabolism, but it also affects the healthiness of your bones. In addition, magnesium helps control blood pressure, regulates the rhythm of your heart, prevents muscle cramps, and improves the action of your insulin, a real bonus for anyone with diabetes or prediabetes.

In fact, low levels of magnesium have been associated with increased blood pressure, insulin resistance, and type 2 diabetes, and low serum levels have been found to be a strong independent predictor of diabetes due to magnesium's facilitation of insulin action and its enzyme activity, which is involved in carbohydrate metabolism. Thus, a magnesium deficiency can interfere with your binding of insulin, uptake of glucose into cells, and glucose use. This was confirmed by a recent study showing that 2.5 grams of a magnesium chloride solution taken daily for 16 weeks improved insulin sensitivity and glycemic control in older people with type 2 diabetes who had previously low levels of serum magnesium.

If your diabetes control is currently less than optimal, you may want to assess your dietary magnesium intake before deciding whether to supplement with this mineral. In people who don't have diabetes, magnesium levels are not normally low, but this mineral, like zinc, can be depleted through excessive urination resulting from poorly controlled diabetes or excessive sweating (such as during exercise); frequent muscle cramps may be one symptom of a deficiency. On the other hand, an excessive intake of magnesium can cause transient diarrhea, but is otherwise safe—except if you have kidney failure, in which case you will need to restrict your intake. You probably shouldn't supplement with more than 350 mg daily, even though higher levels have been taken with minimal side effects. If your diabetes is well controlled, you will not need to supplement your magnesium. Simply increase your intake with healthier food choices, since it is available in such a wide variety of foods.

Chromium. While a deficiency of this mineral in nondiabetic people is rare, if you have diabetes, taking supplements of chromium, alone or in combination with zinc, can improve your glucose tolerance and antioxidant enzyme status. Chromium increases the binding of insulin to receptors in fat and muscle and enhances your total number of insulin receptors and their activity. If your BG levels are normal, extra intake of chromium has minimal effect, but if you are continually hyperglycemic, this mineral may help reduce your BG levels by improving your insulin action.

And its positive effects may not stop there. In one study on elderly adults with type 2 diabetes, chromium supplements of 200 mcg twice daily for three weeks resulted not only in improvements in overall BG levels, but also in a reduction of blood cholesterol levels, an added benefit. Moreover, this mineral may have the capacity to reduce your oxidative stress if your diabetes is poorly controlled (but not if your BG levels are normal). Finally, low chromium levels are associated with a greater risk of heart attack in men, and chromium supplements have recently been found to reduce your risk of developing fatal heart arrhythmias (abnormal beats that can result in your heart stopping altogether) by shortening prolonged **QT intervals** caused by diabetes. The QT interval, which is the time in your heart's contraction cycle when an abnormal rhythm is most likely to begin, is often prolonged when you have diabetes, and this prolongation has been associated with high BG levels, high insulin levels, and reduced sensitivity to insulin.

Chromium can be obtained through meat, organ meats, oysters (a particularly good source), cheese, whole-grain products, asparagus, and beer. If you decide to take a chromium supplement, doses of less than 1,000 mcg per day appear to be safe for short-term use; do not exceed 200 mcg per day if you are taking them over long periods of time. High doses of chromium picolinate can result in toxicity, but newer, improved forms of synthetic chromium that are less toxic are currently being investigated for their therapeutic value.

TIP
40

NO MATTER YOUR WEIGHT

CHROMIUM PICOLINATE supplements have been marketed to athletes and others as a means to increase muscle mass and lose body fat as s de effects of its insulin-sensitizing ability. However, well-designed research studies have not confirmed these claims. If you do choose to take chromium supplements, do it to improve your insulin sensitivity, lower your blood cholesterol, or increase your antioxidant status, *not* to lose weight.

Vanadium and vanadyl salts. Although considered a nonessential nutrient, when taken as vanadyl sulfate, a salt of vanadium, this trace mineral may be able to lower your BG levels by decreasing your liver's production of glucose, along with increasing the insulin sensitivity of your muscles. Through these actions, vanadyl ions may be effective in treating or relieving diabetes and even preventing its onset. Treatment with vanadyl sulfate has also been shown to increase glutathione levels in the kidneys of diabetic rats; thus it is also potentially effective in preventing renal diabetic complications.

Good food sources of vanadium include shellfish, whole-grain products, parsley, mushrooms, and black pepper. The average American diet supplies 15 to 30 mcg of vanadium daily, but since it has not been deemed "essential," no recommended intake has been established. When you take supplements in larger doses, though, you may end up with diarrhea and toxicity. Thus, you should consult with your healthcare provider before starting on vanadium supplements of any sort.

THE BOTTOM LINE ON STEP 6
Make the Most of Meds and Supplements

▶ Diabetic medications are the third cornerstone in effective diabetes management and should not be viewed as the result of a failure on your part to control your BG.

▶ Oral diabetic medications come in a variety of different classes, each with its own unique actions on your body.

▶ Certain oral diabetic medications can increase your risk of hypoglycemia with exercise.

▶ The use of insulin and insulin analogs can effectively meet your body's baseline insulin needs, as well as your requirements for insulin with meals and snacks.

▶ Inhaled and oral insulin choices may soon become available and free you of the need to take insulin injections.

▶ Some other medications may negatively affect your body's response to exercise.

▶ Your body's normal antioxidant defenses are weakened by hyperglycemia, and taking antioxidant supplements may benefit you, especially if your BG is not well controlled.

► Certain vitamins (e.g., vitamin D), minerals (e.g., magnesium), and other nutrients (e.g., cinnamon) may have antidiabetic effects.

► Try to obtain your essential nutrients naturally, through foods, if at all possible; use nutritional supplements only if you're unable to consume enough of them.

Again, if you're not successful in controlling your BG with the first two cornerstones of diabetes management—diet and exercise—alone, please don't feel that you have failed or that you might as well stop trying so hard. Diabetes doesn't occur until your insulin is both less effective (due to insulin resistance) and less abundant (due to beta cell loss), and glycemic control is not always possible without the addition of medications—even with diligent efforts. Be your own advocate and check with your physician or health-care provider about your use of prescribed medications, particularly if your BG levels aren't staying within your target values. In addition, although there simply aren't enough diabetes specialists to go around, be open to the possibility of changing physicians if you're not satisfied with the advice and care that you're getting. The key to preventing diabetic complications is undeniably to optimize your BG control. Focus on controlling your glucose levels through whatever means possible, including a diabetic medication or two or even supplemental insulin, to gain the health benefits of the best possible control.

If you're interested in taking supplements, go back and review what each vitamin or mineral can or can't do for you before deciding which one(s) to take. The best advice for improving your nutrient intake, however, is to start by making as many of the dietary improvements recommended in step 4 and this fitness step as possible. Add in key foods high in antioxidants and other nutrients that diabetes can deplete, such as spinach, broccoli, dark green leafy vegetables, nuts and seeds, sweet potatoes, whole grains, tomatoes, strawberries, peaches, citrus fruits, black pepper, vitamin D—-fortified soy milk, and limited amounts of semisweet, dark chocolate. If you can get yourself to eat more of these foods and fewer highly refined ones, your insulin sensitivity will improve without the need for any supplements.

DIABETES FITNESS PLAN STEP 6
in a Nutshell

EFFECTIVE USE of diabetic and other medications along with certain nutritional supplements may enable you to better control your diabetes and other health problems so that you can live a longer and healthier life.

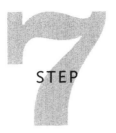

STEP

Stay Motivated for Your Lifetime

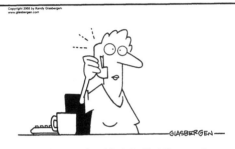

"Welcome to the Diabetic Hotline! If you need a
new excuse for cheating on your diet, press 1. If you
need a new excuse for skipping your workout, press 2..."

YOU MAY HAVE started out with the best of intentions to become more fit, and you may even have invested in some new walking shoes—so why are they still sitting in the box next to your brand-new pair of polyester-blend athletic socks? My expert diagnosis: your fitness motivation needs an overhaul.

There is hope for you yet—you have read through this book all the way to the seventh step, after all. What you need to do now is to muster up the motivation to follow this last and crucial step on your road to diabetes fitness. To find out what you can do to overcome common obstacles to being active and to motivate yourself to make exercise an integral part of your diabetes and health management, read on for some tips guaranteed to get you up off the couch forever.

Take it one day at a time . . . for the rest of your life

The definition of insanity is repeating the same behavior over and over again, but expecting different results every time. You don't have to dramatically change everything about your lifestyle all at once, but effectively preventing and controlling your prediabetes or type 2 diabetes is going to involve doing something differently . . . permanently. The healthy nutritional changes that you implement for yourself should *never* be interpreted as "going on a diet," which implies that the "diet" will end at some point. If you avoid calling your meal plan a "diet," you will have a much more positive attitude toward the changes you make.

Along the same lines, if "exercise" is a bad word around your house, call it "physical activity" or "moving more" or something else with a less negative connotation. Get started by becoming more active throughout the day, and try to sit less and move around or stand more. I guarantee that you won't even realize that what you're doing counts as exercise. Start today, and take it one day at a time.

Lose the diets

If some weight loss is your goal, do yourself a favor and do *not* follow any drastic fad diet or unbalanced diet plan. Since most diets fail at some point if permanent changes are not made, you will likely gain the weight back afterward anyway—unless, of course, you choose to adopt a healthier eating plan and incorporate more physical activity into your life. Just gaining or retaining muscle mass will increase your round-the-clock energy expenditure without you giving it a thought. So, start moving more in any way possible, give up dieting, develop a healthy relationship to eating in general, and live well in spite of diabetes and at any body weight.

TIP

41

NO MATTER YOUR WEIGHT

IF YOU do it regularly, exercise is more likely to help you to lose weight and keep it off than any fad diet you have ever been on. Increasing your muscle mass likewise bumps up your calorie usage all day long. Diets, on the other hand, can cause a reduction in your metabolic rate, particularly if you are taking in fewer than 1,000 calories a day.

Keep reminding yourself that exercise can save your life

Regular exercise can lessen the potential impact of most of your cardiovascular risk factors, including elevated cholesterol levels, insulin resistance, obesity, and hypertension. High blood pressure is associated with higher levels of insulin, and regular physical activity can result in lower blood pressure *and* reduced circulating levels of insulin. If you do nothing but regular walking, it can lengthen your life—as it is likely the best medicine for both the prevention and treatment of type 2 diabetes. Thus, good BG control, if you achieve it with the help of regular physical activity, has the potential to prevent or delay almost all of the potential long-term health complications of diabetes, and it's never too late to get started reaping the health benefits.

Why, then, do so many people still consider "exercise" to be a punishment of some sort to be avoided at all cost? Proofs of this misperception are everywhere. For instance, one group of people composed of 64 male and 112 female Mexicans ages 30 to 75 (with a mean age of 55 years) with type 2 diabetes reported following the correct dose of prescribed diabetes pills or insulin 78 percent of the time, eating recommended food portions over half of the time, and exercising three or more times per week only 44 percent of the time, making exercise the least adhered-to part of their diabetes care plans. Based on other results of that study, your adherence to exercise is likely to be worse if you're depressed or have a history of excessive alcohol intake; more importantly, however, you'll be most likely to follow the recommendations if you are more knowledgeable about diabetes, regularly check your BG at home, have good health, and communicate better with your doctor.

The more you know, the easier you'll find your way to fitness

Thus, it appears that arming yourself with more knowledge about diabetes is the first step to increasing your adherence to better diabetes self-care and to attaining good health—and you have already done that by reading this book. Another step would be to find ways to control your feelings of depression. When you are depressed or in an emotional funk of any sort, the last thing you usually feel motivated to do is anything resembling exercise. The funny thing about physical activity, as we discussed, is that it *lowers* levels of depression and anxiety—so your current sedentary behaviors may actually be contributing to your being depressed! To break this vicious cycle of depression and inactivity and to better motivate yourself in general, follow the tips given in the remainder of this fitness step.

Motivational tips to keep yourself fit

Move more to get more energy. Knowing all that you now know about why exercise is so great for you, why can't you motivate yourself to do it? People complain all the time about being "too tired" to exercise. What you may not realize, though, is that your *lack* of exercise is probably most responsible for making you feel tired. Even active individuals who take a few weeks off from their normal activities begin to feel more sluggish, lethargic, and unmotivated to exercise. The best thing to do in that case is to start moving more. Almost invariably, you will begin to feel more energized rather than less so. For example, when you feel tired, instead of taking a nap, take a short walk; you'll feel the difference the activity makes in your energy levels, and more than likely, it'll recharge your batteries far more than a nap.

Always have a backup plan for exercise. Of course, there are many other barriers to being physically active. It may be as simple as the weather not being conducive to walking outdoors certain days or times of year. You need to have a "Plan B," a backup plan for being active, such as walking in the mall or doing an alternate activity like an exercise video at home that day. Understandably, not everyone has the same exercise opportunities or facilities available. Among certain segments of the population, for example, unaffordable facilities and unavailable child care, high crime rates, fear for personal safety (such as during outdoor walking), and culturally inappropriate activities can act as barriers. Moreover, some individuals lack confidence in their ability to be physically active (especially if they are overweight), while others lack self-management skills or encouragement and support from family members and friends. You may simply be one of those people who lack the self-motivation to become and stay physically active on their own.

Lose the "bad health" excuse. Poor health is another major barrier to exercise participation, but not one that can't be overcome. In fact, becoming more active actually improves your health in many ways; it is simply a misperception that you can't exercise because of your ailing health. Among the elderly, not just poor health, but also age itself may be considered an exercise barrier. But remember that what you don't use, you lose. We are all aging and losing muscle mass as time marches on, but you can fight back and prevent some of the decline just by being physically active. Remember this: most of the diseases that you associate with older age are actually caused by a sedentary lifestyle, not by advancing age, so most of them can be reversed to a large extent by being active. For elderly adults, engaging in a "functional tasks" exercise program may be more effective for maintaining and increasing the ability to perform daily activities than a resistance exercise program.

Make exercise more convenient. Another barrier to exercise is that it is inconvenient, especially when no parks, walking trails, fitness centers, or community recreational centers are located nearby. Likely for that reason, home-based programs appear to be superior to center-based programs in terms of adherence to exercise (especially in the long term) because of the convenience factor—so it may be worthwhile to dust off that stationary bike and bring it out of the basement or attic (or take off the clothes that you have been hanging on it in your bedroom). If nothing else, it'll help you become more time-efficient—you can watch your favorite TV show or movie or catch up on your reading while you bike. An added bonus is that doing such activities during your exercise session will make the time pass more quickly.

If you're lacking the time, exercise one step at a time. Actually, the most common reason adults give for not exercising on a regular basis is lack of time, so being able to do two things at once is important. Moreover, if you can stop thinking of exercise as only planned activities and instead simply try to move more—anytime, anywhere—you will be amazed at how much more active you will become and how little time you will feel you are sacrificing to do it. Any movement you do increases the total amount of energy that you expend in a day. In fact, for most people, the majority of their calorie use during the day comes from unstructured activities (as discussed in step 2) rather than from a formal exercise plan. Managing to take just 2,000 more steps every day can make the difference between additional weight gain and maintaining or losing weight. Wear an inexpensive pedometer as a simple way to motivate yourself to take those steps.

Trick yourself into being more active all day long. It's too bad that motivation is not available in pill form along with directions: "Just take one in the morning and never lack a moment's motivation all day." In reality, motivation comes in many forms, and the easiest way to stay motivated is to simply trick yourself into being more physically active without giving it much thought. That way, your former unmotivated self won't have a chance to convince your new self—the one with the new and improved fitness goals—to revert back to your previous lifestyle.

Trick yourself by doing any of the following activities on a daily basis: if you have a sedentary job, get up and walk around the office, building, or block on your short breaks, and take the stairs instead of the elevator whenever you can. Walk to someone else's office or house to deliver a message instead of relying on the phone or e-mail. Park your car at the far end of the parking lot and walk a little extra to get to your destination. (Stop being one of those people who will wait ten minutes for a spot up close to open up when they could have just parked a little farther away and walked there faster instead.) Your activities don't have to be done at a high intensity to be effective.

Tips for Keeping Your Exercise Motivation Strong

▶ Get yourself an exercise buddy (or even a dog who needs to be walked).

▶ Use sticker charts or other motivational tools to track your progress.

▶ Schedule structured exercise into your day on your calendar or "To Do" list.

▶ Break your larger goals into smaller, realistic stepping stones (e.g., daily and weekly physical activity goals).

▶ Reward yourself for meeting your goals with noncaloric treats or outings.

▶ Plan to do fun physical activities that you really enjoy as often as possible.

▶ Wear a pedometer (at least occasionally) as a reminder to take more daily steps.

▶ Have a backup plan that includes alternate activities in case of inclement weather or other barriers to your planned exercise.

▶ Distract yourself while you exercise by reading a book or magazine, watching TV, listening to music or a book on tape, or talking with a friend.

▶ Don't start out exercising too intensely or you're likely to get discouraged or injured.

▶ If you get out of your normal routine and are having trouble getting restarted, simply take small steps in that direction.

Check around for fun activities in your community. As far as becoming more involved in structured exercise programs, check around to find out what exercise programs are located in your workplace or nearby in your community. You can often find groups of individuals who walk together during lunch breaks, or you may be able to join a low-impact aerobics or other exercise class offered at your workplace or a nearby recreation center. Other activity programs that you may not be aware of might be available in your area, including formal or informal dance classes through community centers or other recreation-oriented groups. In some regions of the country (such as Louisiana and Virginia), mobile gyms based out of an equipped RV are now being funded and taken around for weekly use by older people and other underserved populations in lower-income areas to give them access to exercise equipment that they would not likely have otherwise.

Get yourself a reliable exercise buddy, or bring the whole family along. There's no need to go it alone. Having a regular (and reliable) exercise buddy increases your likelihood of showing up (since someone else is counting on you to be there) and also makes your activities more socially oriented. Get your spouse, other family members, friends, and coworkers to join in your physical activities, especially during your leisure time, as having a good social network to support your exercise habit will help your adherence over the long run. Across all cultures, ages, and sexes, social support from family, peers, communities, and health-care providers results in modest improvements in exercise motivation and adherence. Even people with diabetes living in rural settings in the Midwest are reportedly more likely to exercise regularly if their physicians help them devise plans to increase their daily exercise and then follow up with them to keep them on track.

Keep track of your progress, and reward yourself. If you have already started an exercise program and are having trouble keeping it up (especially if you've previously been one of those 50 percent of people who drop out within the first six months), there are a few things that you can do to keep yourself motivated. Set realistic exercise goals or milestones to keep track of your hard work, and set up rewards for yourself when you meet them. Who says that stickers and treats are just for kids? If it works for you, use a sticker chart or some other visible record of physical activities that you accomplish each day and then give yourself frequent reinforcement with "tokens" or "treats" (preferably noncaloric ones) when you meet your goals. Maybe you can promise yourself an outing to somewhere special, the purchase of a coveted item, or anything else that is reasonable and effectively motivates you to exercise. Helpful recommendations for physical activities, activity logs, and other motivational tools are also widely available.

Put your exercise down on your calendar. Never make the mistake of assuming that structured exercise will happen just because you claim that you want to do it a certain number of days per week or month. Actually *schedule* the exercise by writing it down in your agenda or calendar as you would for other appointments or activities. Break up your larger goals into stepping-stone goals, by the day, week, and month, and if you miss one of your goals, try to make the rest of them happen anyway. Making exercise goals less concrete and open-ended (like saying that you are going to exercise three times a week without trying to schedule the days in advance) often sets you up for failure.

Keep it simple, make it fun, and mix it up. Once exercise becomes an integrated part of your lifestyle, you're much more likely to maintain it permanently. To increase your long-term compliance, your exercise plan should be as uncomplicated as possible, geared toward your unique health needs, beliefs, and goals, and enjoyable. People commonly complain about exercise being boring. While many adults may force themselves to exercise solely for the health benefits (honestly, most of them may not really like to exercise that much), no one is saying that it couldn't or shouldn't be enjoyable. In reality, most adults need exercise to be fun, too, or they lose their motivation to do it over time. To prevent boredom with your exercise program, try varying your exercise frequently—both what you do and how hard or long you do it. Knowing that you don't have to do the same workout day after day is very motivating. Also, try to at least occasionally pick activities that you truly enjoy, such as dancing or golf (as long as you walk and carry your own clubs). Realistically, would you actually adhere to an exercise program that reminds you of the one depicted in Gary Larson's cartoon "Aerobics in Hell" (Okay! Five million leg lifts, right leg first! Ready, set!)? Have fun with your exercise to more easily make it a permanent and integral part of your diabetes management.

Distract yourself during workouts. Along the same lines, there is absolutely nothing wrong with using every means at your disposal to distract yourself while you exercise to make the time go by more quickly and less painfully. On days you can't exercise with someone else or get outside, walk in place while you read a book or magazine (this also works on your balance) or watch a movie or your favorite TV program (or better yet, tape your shows first and then fast forward through all the boring commercials). If you prefer audio distractions, listen to music, your favorite radio show, or books on tape during your workouts, or use your exercise time to catch up on your long phone calls. If you're like most people, just having someone to talk with during your activities can make them pass much more quickly—which is another reason to recruit an exercise buddy (or two).

Don't make your workouts too hard. Another point to remember is that the opposite of fun is agony. Don't start out exercising too intensely, or it will be too hard and unenjoyable (particularly if it ends up making you really sore for a few days afterward). In such a case, human nature will prevail, and you will find excuses not to do it again. Additionally, you are more likely to injure yourself if your exercise intensity is too high to start. Use the Talk Test as your guide: if you can't comfortably carry on a conversation with someone else while you are exercising, then you are working harder than necessary to achieve your fitness and health goals. Simply slow down and focus instead on exercising a little bit longer instead of burning out your desire to be active.

If you fall off the wagon, get back on. There will undoubtedly be days when you want to forget you have diabetes or prediabetes and chuck all your lifestyle changes out the window—believe me, we all have days like that. Part of being more fit is learning how to conquer your resistance to change and finding your way back to a healthier way of living if you do get off track. Always keep the memory of how much better you felt when you made the changes to use as motivation when you need to. If you find yourself falling off the exercise "wagon" in either minor or major ways, forgive yourself for your lapse and get back on. A short break from your normal routine—such as for vacations, illness or injuries, or other changes in your normal schedule—does not mean that you can't start scheduling your physical activity back in again. During any break, be it short or long, try to keep up all of your extra movement during the day even if you can't manage to do anything else; at least that way you will be less likely to lose any fitness gains that you have made so far, which will make it easier to get back into doing more as quickly as possible.

Start the wagon up slowly. When you begin exercising, or if you're starting back after a lapse, remember that you may need to begin at a lower intensity (i.e., lighter weights, less resistance, or a slower walking speed) to avoid burnout, muscle soreness, or even injury. Even doing only 5 to 10 minutes at a time (instead of 30 or more minutes) is fine. If you really don't want to exercise, make a deal with yourself that you will only do it for 5 or 10 minutes to get yourself started (which is often the hardest part); once you are actually up and moving, you may actually start to feel good enough to go past the time you tricked yourself into doing. The key is to just begin anew using any means possible.

THE BOTTOM LINE ON STEP 7
Stay Motivated for Your Lifetime

► Your lifestyle changes need not be drastic, but they do have to become permanent.

► Lose your "bad health" excuse for not exercising more.

► Trick yourself into exercise by simply moving more throughout the day.

► Put your more structured activities down on your calendar, keep track of your progress, and reward yourself for meeting your goals.

► Recruit an exercise buddy or two to join in the fun.

► Find ways to distract yourself during workouts to make the time pass more quickly.

► Don't start out working too hard, or you'll likely injure yourself or decide to quit.

► Remember to keep your physical activities convenient, enjoyable, and varied to prevent excuses to avoid doing it.

► If you fall off the exercise wagon, get back on it as soon as you can, but start back slowly.

While a lot of this last step to diabetes fitness may sound like common sense, it is vitally important. Without the motivation to move more, eat better, control your stress, and take your prescribed medications, it will be almost impossible for you to reach your goals and effectively control your diabetes. It's all about feeling good while you still have a life left to live, which I am convinced can only be accomplished through these diabetes fitness steps. You have much more to gain—both physically and mentally—by becoming fit than you may actually realize, and it is *never* too late to start.

DIABETES FITNESS PLAN STEP 7
in a Nutshell

MOTIVATION TO exercise comes in many forms. Try out different strategies until you find the ones that work for you to make healthy lifestyle changes that will last for the rest of your long and healthy life.

Follow the Steps
to Diabetes Fitness

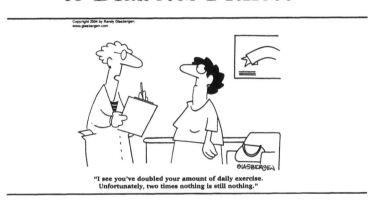

"I see you've doubled your amount of daily exercise.
Unfortunately, two times nothing is still nothing."

As you have learned throughout this book, "fitness" means many things for a person with diabetes or insulin resistance. Insulin resistance may be the hallmark of prediabetes and type 2 diabetes, but it is by no means the only health-related problem. Of the three diabetes management cornerstones—diet, medications, and exercise—assuredly the one with the greatest potential for a positive impact on your diabetes control and your overall health is exercise.

Nothing does it better than exercise

The superlative benefits of any form of physical activity come from the fact that it can lessen the impact of multiple health concerns simultaneously. Visceral fat stored within your abdomen is by far the most deleterious type of body fat in terms of your metabolic function, but as you have learned in this book, both moderate aerobic exercise and resistance training (done even only twice a week) result in losses of visceral fat that dieting alone does not. Moreover, it's entirely possible to be fit regardless of your body weight and gain almost all of the associated health benefits *without* struggling to lose weight and keep it off. Regular physical activity of any kind can even prevent you from developing type 2 diabetes in the first place or reverse prediabetes, even if your "bad" genes put you at higher risk for either health condition. Even though exercise can't prevent type 1 diabetes, it can prevent type 1.5 diabetes ("double diabetes") by reversing or preventing insulin resistance in people who have type 1, making it easier for them (myself included) to effectively control their BG levels and prevent diabetic complications.

Your diet still matters

That is not to say that if you exercise regularly, you will not benefit from making some changes to your diet—you absolutely will. Your overall fitness can be significantly increased by the addition of more fiber to your daily food intake and the subtraction of highly refined food products. Physical activity will allow you to be a little more slack in the diet department and still do well with your BG control, but only up to a point. Even one of the original running gurus, Jim Fixx, an avid marathoner, ended up dying from a massive heart attack while running—and at a relatively young age—primarily due to his failure to make heart-healthy changes to his diet, even though he knew that his cholesterol levels were high and his family history of heart disease strong. Diabetes is not just a carbohydrate-processing disorder; it is also a disorder of lipids—blood fats—that contributes to the development of plaque formation in arteries and circulatory problems throughout your body. Your food intake can affect your glucose levels *and* your blood fats, as can your exercise habits.

Medications can save your life

If I hadn't been taking insulin for the past thirty-seven years, I wouldn't be here to write this book for you. Likewise, you would be remiss to scoff at the third cornerstone of diabetes management: medications. Despite their potential negative side effects, effective use of prescribed medications can promote better health with diabetes via improved BG control and lower circulating levels of cholesterol and other blood fats. In addition, such medications may assist you in staving off any number of diabetes-related complications that can reduce the quality and length of your life. Modify your lifestyle for the better first (every aspect of your health will undoubtedly benefit), but what diet and exercise can't fix, leave to the pharmaceuticals.

As for other nutritional supplements, your need for them mostly depends on your diet, so eat well to limit your potential for developing any vitamin and mineral deficiencies that would upset your metabolic balance or contribute to the development of diabetic complications. Magnesium deficiencies—common with diabetes—are a good example, as low levels of that essential mineral can worsen control of hypertension, diabetes, and a number of other metabolic processes that can accelerate heart disease.

Adding in a fourth cornerstone

Finally, it is my professional (and personal) opinion that a fourth cornerstone should be added to the first three: stress management. I know from personal experience that going through your life with a chronic health problem (or several simultaneously) is absolutely no fun. Living with diabetes is a daily challenge, and it requires your attention 24 hours a day, seven days a week, 365 days a year. You can't leave home and take a vacation from it (at least, not without suffering some physical consequences), and it is always there, hovering in the background, threatening to ruin your day even when everything else is going right. So, if you can't beat it, the best thing to do is to live well with it. This includes dealing effectively with the stress that having diabetes causes and the effect that stress from any source has on your BG levels, lessening your feelings of depression, and improving your self-image and self-esteem.

The first three management cornerstones can help you deal with the unofficial fourth one, and, not surprisingly, physical activity again leads the pack in lessening the emotional implications of living with diabetes. Regardless of whether diabetes leads to depression or depression actually begets diabetes, regular physical activity can lessen the impact of either one. It also helps you sleep better, which can prevent elevations in cortisol levels that can contribute to both physical and emotional problems.

The goal of this entire book has been to lead you through what I know from both professional and personal experience are the seven crucial steps to achieving fitness with diabetes, no matter your body size or weight, and without a diet in sight. Although diabetes, prediabetes, and insulin resistance will likely always remain a part of your vocabulary, achieving "diabetes fitness" to live well for the rest of your long life is truly the best revenge.

The 7 Step Diabetes Fitness Plan Recap

Step 1: Your lifestyle choices matter most in controlling your diabetes or prediabetes. The goal is to improve your insulin sensitivity and glucose use, and physical activity and increased fitness are best suited to help you accomplish this goal, no matter how much you weigh.

Step 2: Regardless of your current physical condition, there are myriad easy and effective ways to start moving more to make the undeniable benefits of increased physical activity on your diabetes control and general health yours to keep for the rest of your life.

Step 3: Your physical fitness and diabetes control will benefit most from a varied exercise program that includes aerobic exercise of differing intensities, resistance training, regular stretching, body "core" exercises, and a weekly day of rest.

Step 4: Optimal eating is just as vital to diabetes fitness as physical activity as the two work in concert. Stick with natural, colorful, high-fiber, low-GI foods and smaller portions to control your diabetes and your body weight.

Step 5: Your emotional health is just as important as your physical health when it comes to effectively controlling your diabetes and preventing loss of quality of life from depression, dementia, or disordered eating. Physical activity can help you conquer them all.

Step 6: Effective use of diabetic and other medications along with certain nutritional supplements may enable you to better control your diabetes and other health problems so that you can live a longer and healthier life.

Step 7: Motivation to exercise comes in many forms. Try out different strategies until you find the ones that work for you to make healthy lifestyle changes that will last for the rest of your long and healthy life.

Target Heart Rate Training Zones for Optimal Fitness

R HR = RESTING heart rate, which you should optimally measure first thing in the morning before you eat, drink, or move around. Heart Rate (HR) values are estimated as a target zone of 50 to 85 percent of your heart rate reserve (HRR). Your HRR is simply the difference between your highest and lowest HRs (i.e., your estimated maximal HR minus your RHR). To find a target range, multiply your HRR by 50 percent for the low end and by 85 percent for the highest value. The table gives you those ranges based on the median age for each range.

AGE

RHR	15-19	20-24	25-29	30-34	35-39	40-44	45-49	50-54	55-59	60-64	65-69	70-74	75-79	80-84	85-89	90-94	95-99
45-49	125-180	123-175	120-171	118-167	115-163	113-158	110-154	108-150	105-146	103-141	100-137	98-133	95-128	93-124	90-120	88-116	85-111
50-54	127-181	125-176	122-172	120-168	117-164	115-159	112-155	110-151	107-147	105-142	102-138	100-134	97-129	95-125	92-121	90-117	87-112
55-59	130-181	128-176	125-172	123-168	120-164	118-159	115-155	113-151	110-147	108-142	105-138	103-134	100-129	98-125	95-121	93-117	90-112
60-64	132-182	130-177	127-173	125-169	122-165	120-160	117-156	115-152	112-148	110-143	107-139	105-135	102-130	100-126	97-122	95-118	92-113
65-69	135-183	133-178	130-174	128-170	125-166	123-161	120-157	118-153	115-149	113-144	110-140	108-136	105-131	103-127	100-123	98-119	95-114
70-74	137-184	135-179	132-175	130-171	127-167	125-162	122-158	120-154	117-150	115-145	112-141	110-137	107-132	105-128	102-124	100-120	97-115
75-79	140-184	138-180	135-176	133-172	130-168	128-163	125-159	123-155	120-151	118-146	115-142	113-138	110-133	108-129	105-125	103-121	100-116
80-84	142-185	140-181	137-177	135-173	132-169	130-164	127-160	125-156	122-152	120-147	117-143	115-139	112-134	110-130	107-126	105-122	102-117
85-89	145-186	143-181	140-177	138-173	135-169	133-164	130-160	128-156	125-152	123-147	120-143	118-139	115-134	113-130	110-126	108-122	105-117
90-94	148-186	145-182	142-178	140-174	138-170	135-165	132-161	130-157	128-153	125-148	122-144	120-140	118-135	115-131	112-127	110-123	108-118
95-99	150-187	148-183	145-179	143-175	140-171	138-166	135-162	133-158	130-154	128-149	125-145	123-140	120-136	118-132	115-128	113-124	110-119

Glycemic Index Values and Glycemic Load of Common Foods

(PER 50-GRAM SERVING)

I NFORMATION IN PARENTHESES represents glycemic index and glycemic load, respectively. GI is based on a standard serving of 50 grams of digestible carbohydrate, while the product of a food's GI and its total available carbohydrate content in a "typical" serving represents its GL. The GI value is based on a comparison to glucose, which has a GI value of 100. Information from the International Table of Glycemic Index and Load Values: 2002.

	LOW GI (<55)	MEDIUM GI (55 to 70)	HIGH GI (>70)
LOW GL **(< 10)**	Apples (38,6) Beans, baked (48,7) Beans, kidney (28,7) Bread, whole-grain (51,7) Carrots (47,3) Cereal, All-Bran (42,9) Chickpeas (28,8) Cookie, oatmeal (54,9) Fructose sweetener (20,2) Grapefruit (25,3) Grapes (46,8) Ice cream, low-fat (43,5) Ice cream, premium (38,4) Juice, carrot (43,10) Juice, tomato (38,4) Lentils, red (26,5) M&M's, peanut (33,6) Milk, skim (32,4)	Apricots (57,5) Beets (64,5) Cantaloupe (65,4) Honey (55,10) Ice cream, regular (61,8) Peaches, canned in heavy syrup (55,9) Pineapple (59,7) 7-grain bread (55,8) Sugar, white (68,7)	Bread, white flour (70,10) Bread, whole-wheat (71,9) Glucose (99,10) Popcorn (72,8) Watermelon (72,4)

	LOW GI (<55)	MEDIUM GI (55 to 70)	HIGH GI (>70)
LOW GL (< 10)	Milk, soy (42,7) Milk, whole (40,3) Oranges (42,5) Peaches (42,5) Peaches, canned in juice (38,9) Peanuts (14,1) Pears (38,4) Peas, green (48,3) Prunes (29,10) Strawberries (40,1) Tortellini, cheese (50,10) Yogurt, low-fat (27,7) Yogurt, nonfat, artificially sweetened (24,3)		
MEDIUM GL (11 to 19)	Bananas (52,12) Beans, navy (38,12) Bread, sourdough wheat (54,15) Buckwheat (54,16) Cookie bar, Twix (44,17) Corn, sweet (53,17) Fettuccine (40,18) Juice, apple (40,12) Juice, grapefruit (48,11) Juice, pineapple (46,16) Ravioli, meat (39,15)	Cake, angel food (67,19) Cereal, Raisin Bran (61,12) Cereal, Special K (69,14) Croissant (67,17) Juice, orange (57,15) Muffin, bran (60,15) Oatmeal, old-fashioned (58,13) Oatmeal, quick (66,17) Pizza, cheese (60,16) Potatoes, new (57,12) Potatoes, sweet (61,17) Rice, brown, boiled (55,18) Rice, wild (57,18)	Doughnut, cake-type (76,17) Cereal, Cheerios (74,15) Cereal, Grape Nuts (75,16) Cereal, shredded wheat (75,15) Cereal, Total (76,17) Crackers, soda (74,12) Gatorade, 12 oz. (78,17) Potatoes, mashed (85,17) Pretzels (83,16) Muffin, English (77,11) Rice cakes, puffed (78, 17) Wafers, vanilla (77,14)
HIGH GL (> 20)	Linguine (46,22) Macaroni (47,23) Spaghetti (44,21)	Candy bar, Mars (65,26) Candy bar, Snickers (68,23) Coca-Cola, 12 oz. can (63,23) Cranberry juice cocktail (68,24) Couscous (65,23) Kudos, whole-grain bar, chocolate chip (62,20) Macaroni and cheese, boxed (64,32) Power Bar (56,24) Raisins (64,28) Rice, white, boiled (64,23)	Bagel, white flour (72,25) Candy, Skittles (70,32) Cereal, cornflakes (92,24) Cereal, Golden Grahams (71,18) Cereal, Krispix (87,22) Cereal, Rice Krispies (82,22) French fries (75,22) Fruit bars, strawberry (90,23) Fruit roll-ups (99,24) Jelly beans (78,22) Potato, baked (85,26) Pop Tart, double chocolate (70,24)

APPENDIX D

General Nutrition and Shopping Guide

CONSUME FREELY	LIMIT CONSUMPTION OF	AVOID WHENEVER POSSIBLE
Water; noncaloric drinks; diet, non-cola, caffeine-free soda	Diet, caffeinated sodas; regular iced tea; sports drinks	Regular sodas, especially colas; sugary noncarbonated drinks
Fresh raw vegetables; plain frozen vegetables	Vegetables grilled in oil or butter; highly salted vegetables; processed tomato sauces	Canned vegetables; vegetables with added sauces (cream, butter); battered, fried vegetables
Whole fruits; dried fruits (in small portions); canned fruits in natural juices (drained)	100% fruit juices (except apple and white grape); dried fruits with added sweeteners	Fruit "drinks" and "cocktails"; apple and white grape juices; canned fruits in heavy syrup
Whole-grain products (brown rice, oats, barley, etc.); sweet potatoes	Whole-wheat products (bread, crackers, bagels, pasta)	White-flour products (most crackers, doughnuts, breads, cakes, pastries, cookies); white potatoes
Products with no added sugars (and no unhealthy fats)	Products with small amounts of added sugars	Products with large amounts of added sugars
Old-fashioned oatmeal; high-fiber, low-sugar cereals	Quick oats with added sugar; cereals with moderate sugar	Highly processed breakfast cereals full of added sugar
Low-GI, -GL carbohydrates	Moderate-GI, -GL carbohydrates	High-GI, -GL carbohydrates
Unsalted nuts; olive oil; canola oil; monounsaturated fat; liquid vegetable oils; cold-water fish	Salted nuts; reduced-fat margarine; polyunsaturated fat	Saturated fat; trans fat; butter or margarine; hydrogenated or partially hydrogenated oils

CONSUME FREELY	LIMIT CONSUMPTION OF	AVOID WHENEVER POSSIBLE
Nonfat skim milk, ½% or 1% dairy products	Low-fat (2%) or part-skim dairy products	Whole-milk dairy products; cream
Ground turkey breast; skinless chicken and turkey breast; fish (not breaded or fried); legumes	Lean cuts of beef and pork; nonfat hot dogs and lunch meat; turkey bacon; breaded, baked chicken breast (e.g., nuggets)	Steak; ground hamburger; bacon; sausage; hot dogs; regular lunch meat; fatty regular lunch meat; fatty cuts of beef and pork; fried chicken (breaded or with skin on)
Steamed, broiled, or baked foods	Foods grilled in oil, butter, or margarine	Fried foods
Dark, semisweet chocolate	Regular chocolate; peanut M&M's; sugar-free candies	Sugary hard or other candy; Fruit Roll-Ups; Froot Snacks
Low-calorie, nutrient-dense foods	Medium-calorie foods with some nutrients	High-calorie, nutrient-poor foods

Related Web Sites

American Council on Exercise (ACE) (health & fitness tips, fitness Q&A)
http://www.acefitness.org/fitfacts/

American Diabetes Association (ADA) (diabetes information, links, bookstore)
Home page: http://www.diabetes.org/
Club Ped (pedometer walking club) http://www.diabetes.org/ClubPed/index.jsp

American Dietetic Association (nutrition information for consumers)
http://www.eatright.org/Public/

American Obesity Association (obesity information, advocacy, and statistics)
http://www.obesity.org/

America on the Move (national initiative to improve health and quality of life)
http://www.americaonthemove.org/

Beating Diabetes (exercise resources, support, and online personal training)
http://www.beatingdiabetes.org/

Calories Per Hour.Com (physical activity and metabolic calculators and information)
http://www.caloriesperhour.com/

Center for Nutrition Policy and Promotion (CNPP) (nutrition policy, healthy eating index)
Home page: http://www.cnpp.usda.gov/
Interactive Healthy Eating Index and Physical Activity Tool

Center for Science in the Public Interest (*Nutrition Action* newsletter and other information)
http://www.cspinet.org/

Centers for Disease Control and Prevention (CDC) (U.S. government agency)
Diabetes facts: http://www.cdc.gov/health/diabetes.htm

Overweight and obesity facts:
http://www.cdc.gov/nccdphp/dnpa/obesity/index.htm

Diabetes and Wellness Foundation (in partnership with the President's Council on Physical Fitness and Sports)
http://www.diabetesandwellness.org/index.htm

Diabetes Exercise and Sports Association (DESA) (activity-related diabetes organization)
http://www.diabetes-exercise.org/

Diabetes Health magazine (research updates, educational articles, product guides)
http://www.diabeteshealth.com/

Diabetes in Control.com (weekly diabetes research updates)
http://www.diabetesincontrol.com/

Disabled Sports USA (sports information for people with disabilities, including vision loss)
http://www.dsusa.org/

dLife—For Your Diabetes Life (multimedia diabetes information, advocacy, and interaction)
http://dlife.com/

Eating Well: The Magazine of Food and Health (nutrition articles and healthy recipes)
http://www.eatingwell.com/index.htm

Glycemic Index Information and Database (glycemic index information)
http://www.glycemicindex.com/

IDEA Health & Fitness Association (fitness articles and personal trainer locator service)
http://www.ideafit.com/

Joslin Diabetes Center (prominent diabetes treatment center in Boston, nutrition guidelines)
Home page: http://www.joslin.org/
Nutritional guidelines for type 2s:
http://www.joslin.org/Files/Nutrition_ClinGuide.pdf

Just Move.Org (fitness center, progress tracker by the American Heart Association)
http://www.justmove.org/

National Center on Physical Activity and Disability (NCPAD) (lifetime sports with disabilities)
http://www.ncpad.org/

National Institutes of Health (NIH) (U.S. government health agency)
Body mass index (BMI) calculator:
http://www.nhlbisupport.com/bmi/bmicalc.htm
Facts about dietary supplements: http://www.cc.nih.gov/ccc/supplements/
Interactive menu planner: http://hin.nhlbi.nih.gov/menuplanner/menu.cgi
Senior health information (all topics): http://nihseniorhealth.gov/

National Sports Center for the Disabled (NSCD) (sports events information for disabled persons)
http://www.nscd.org/

National Weight Control Registry (successful weight-loss registry and information)
http://www.uchsc.edu/nutrition/WyattJortberg/nwcr.htm

Nutridiary (free online food and exercise diary, food nutrient database)
http://www.nutridiary.com/

Nutrition Data (nutrition data by food item, nutrient density, calorie counter)
http://www.nutritiondata.com/

Reflective Happiness (free happiness index, depression scale, and signature-strengths surveys)
http://www.reflectivehappiness.com/

Shape Up America! (nonprofit group dedicated to achieving a healthy weight for life)
http://www.shapeup.org/

Sheri Colberg's Web site (links to diabetes books, exercise articles, interviews, and more)
http://www.shericolberg.com

Taking Control of Your Diabetes (nonprofit seminars and diabetes information)
http://www.tcoyd.org/

The Diabetes Mall (diabetes supplies and helpful information on pumps, gadgets, and more)
http://www.diabetesnet.com/

The President's Challenge (U.S. government physical activity and fitness awards program)
http://www.presidentschallenge.org/

The President's Council on Physical Fitness and Sports (U.S. government fitness council)
http://www.fitness.gov/

Tufts University Nutrition Navigator (ratings guide to nutrition Web sites)
http://navigator.tufts.edu/

U.S. Department of Agriculture (USDA) (food guide pyramid, food databases)
Food/nutrient database: http://www.nal.usda.gov/fnic/foodcomp/srch/search.htm
New food guide pyramid (2005): http://www.mypyramid.gov/

U.S. Department of Health and Human Services (online brochure on new 2005 dietary guidelines entitled "Finding Your Way to a Healthier You")
http://www.health.gov/dietaryguidelines/dga2005/document/pdf/brochure.pdf

U.S. Food and Drug Administration (FDA) (medications and supplement regulatory agency)
Dietary supplements: http://www.cfsan.fda.gov/~dms/supplmnt.html
Mercury levels in fish: http://www.cfsan.fda.gov/~dms/admehg3.html

Weight-Control Information Network (WIN) (NIH-provided science-based information on weight control, obesity, physical activity, and related nutritional issues)

http://win.niddk.nih.gov/index.htm

Glossary

1-REP MAX: One-repetition maximum, or absolute **muscular strength** on a **resistance training** exercise determined as the maximal weight you can handle just one time before becoming fatigued.

ABDOMINAL OBESITY: Excess weight gain around the waist leading to an "apple" body shape, known for its negative **metabolic** effects.

ACE INHIBITORS: A class of prescribed medications used to treat high blood pressure and early signs of kidney disease.

ADDED SUGARS: Any simple **carbohydrates** (particularly **sucrose** or **dextrose**, which are two names for table sugar) added to foods rather than occurring naturally.

ADENOSINE TRIPHOSPHATE (ATP): The most basic energy compound found in the body; it is used to directly fuel muscle contractions, cellular work, and other **metabolic** processes.

ADIPONECTIN: A **hormone** released by **adipose** cells that influences **insulin** action in the body, as well as the **metabolism** of **lipids** and **glucose**.

ADIPOSE: Body tissues comprised of **fat** cells that act to store excess calories in the form of **triglycerides**.

ADRENALINE: A **hormone** released by the body in response to physical or mental stress and involved in the "flight or fight" syndrome; aka epinephrine.

AEROBIC: Refers to any process in the body that utilizes the **oxygen system** to provide energy.

ALPHA-GLUCOSIDASE INHIBITORS: A class of **oral diabetic medication**s taken with meals to slow the absorption of carbohydrates from the gut, thus reducing the postmeal BG peak.

ALPHA LIPOIC ACID (ALA): A compound found naturally in foods that can also be synthesized by your body and that works with **glutathione** as part of an important **antioxidant** enzyme system to squelch **free radicals** and prevent damage to DNA in cells.

ALZHEIMER'S DISEASE: A progressive disease in which nerve cells in your brain become damaged and brain matter shrinks, resulting in impaired thinking, behavior, and memory.

AMERICAN COLLEGE OF SPORTS MEDICINE (ACSM): The largest American organization dealing with physical activity and medical issues that certifies exercise professionals (e.g., **exercise physiologists**) and makes exercise recommendations to the public.

AMERICAN DIABETES ASSOCIATION (ADA): The largest American medical organization for professionals and the public alike that deals with **diabetes** and related health issues.

AMYLIN: A **hormone** released by the **beta cells** of the **pancreas** along with **insulin** that serves to lower post-meal **BG** levels by slowing the digestion of **glucose** and causing satiety.

ANAEROBIC: Refers to any process in the body that does not use oxygen to provide energy, instead relying on the **phosphagens** or **lactic acid system**.

ANGINA: Chest pain related to reduced **coronary** artery blood flow to the heart due to partial or total blockage from **plaque** or a blood clot.

ANGIOTENSIN II RECEPTOR BLOCKERS (ARBS): A class of prescribed medications used primarily to treat high blood pressure.

ANOREXIA NERVOSA: An **eating disorder** characterized by self-starvation, abnormally low body weight, and poor **self-esteem** that usually requires medical intervention to treat.

ANTIOXIDANT: A substance in the body capable of removing **free radicals** that can cause damage.

ARTIFICIAL SWEETENERS: Synthetically altered compounds that taste sweet like sugar, but that have few or no calories or **carbohydrates**. You can use them in place of other sweeteners to reduce your calorie and/or **carbohydrate** intake and lower the GI value of your foods.

AUTOIMMUNITY: Any disease caused by your body's misguided destruction of its own tissues with your own immune system, such as **type**

1 **diabetes**, rheumatoid arthritis, myasthenia gravis, and other serious chronic diseases.

AUTONOMIC NEUROPATHY: Nerve damage resulting in loss of central nerve function that can cause an abnormally high resting heart rate, a blunted heart rate response to exercise, **orthostatic hypotension, gastroparesis**, and other conditions.

BETA-CAROTENE: A precursor of vitamin A that your body can convert to the active vitamin as needed from food sources such as yellow-orange vegetables.

BETA CELLS: Specialized cells in the **pancreas** that contain the islets of Langerhans—capable of producing both **insulin** and **amylin**.

BIGUANIDES: A class of **oral diabetic medications** that lower **fasting BG** levels and improve **insulin** action in both the liver and muscles.

BLOOD GLUCOSE (BG): The main simple **carbohydrate** found in your circulation, usually expressed in **mg/dl** (United States) or **mM** (everywhere outside the United States). Normal **fasting** levels are 70 to 100 mg/dl.

BODY MASS INDEX (BMI): A metric ratio of your weight in kilograms divided by your height in meters squared. To use pounds and inches instead, insert your values and multiply the number you get by 703 to determine if you are of normal weight, **overweight**, or **obese**.

BULIMIA NERVOSA: An **eating disorder** characterized by periods of binge-purge behavior, with purging accomplished through vomiting, diuretic use, and excessive exercise.

CALCITRIOL: The active form of vitamin D, which can be formed in your skin with adequate exposure to the UV rays in sunlight.

CARBOHYDRATE: A nutrient found in foods composed of sugar units, including simple carbohydrates (**monosaccharides glucose** and **fructose**), **disaccharides** (such as **sucrose**), or **polysaccharides** (**glucose** polymers and starches, such as those found in potatoes). Carbohydrates also exist in your body primarily as **glucose** or **glycogen**.

CARDIOVASCULAR DISEASE: A buildup of **plaque** in arteries that supply blood to your heart, brain, lower limbs, and other areas of your body that can result in **heart attacks, stroke, peripheral vascular disease**, and more.

CHOLESTEROL: A fatty compound essential to your body, but which can, in excessive amounts, contribute to arterial **plaque** formation and **cardiovascular disease**.

COMBINATION THERAPY: Use of two or more **oral diabetic medications** simultaneously in an attempt to achieve **glycemic** control when single therapies are failing to do so.

CONCENTRIC: A muscular contraction that usually occurs during the "lifting" phase of a specific exercise, such as when a weight is moved against the force of gravity (for example, by pushing, pulling, or pressing) and muscles are actively shortening.

COOL-DOWN: A five- to ten-minute period of easier exercise done at the end of more intense physical activity that serves to ease your body's transition to a resting state.

CORONARY: Related to the heart muscle, as in the coronary arteries that supply blood to the heart muscle itself. Sometimes people refer to a heart attack as a "coronary."

CORTISOL: A **hormone** released in response to stress (physical or mental) that mobilizes **fats** and **proteins**, increases **insulin resistance**, and spares **BG**, as during overnight **fasting**.

CROSS TRAINING: Training by doing a wide variety of different sports and physical activities with the purpose of increasing your overall fitness level and preventing **overuse injuries**.

DEHYDRATION: A reduction in normal levels of body fluids due to inadequate fluid intake, excessive sweating, polyuria (excessive urination due to **hyperglycemia**), or a combination of these. Dehydration of just 1 to 2 percent can negatively affect your exercise.

DELAYED-ONSET MUSCLE SORENESS (DOMS): Mild to severe muscle soreness 24 to 48 hours after exercise due to excessive **eccentric** contractions, resulting in local damage to contractile **proteins** in muscle, **inflammation**, swelling, and localized pain.

DEMENTIA: Loss of mental functions, such as thinking, memory, and reasoning, severe enough to interfere with your daily functioning; may be reversible when caused by drugs, alcohol, **hormone** or vitamin imbalances, or **depression**.

DEPRESSION: A mood disorder that causes you to feel sad or hopeless for an extended period of time and that can have a significant impact on your enjoyment of life and your health.

DEXTROSE: Another name for white table sugar.

DIABETES: A **metabolic** disorder affecting insulin release and/or use and levels of **BG** (and often blood **fats**) that can cause serious long-term health complications and early mortality.

DIABETIC COMPLICATIONS: Long-term damage to body tissues due to

hyperglycemia and **oxidative stress** and resulting in health conditions such as **neuropathy, retinopathy, nephropathy**, erectile dysfunction, and **cardiovascular disease**.

DIALYSIS: A medical procedure used to cleanse waste from your blood by filtering it manually when your kidneys stop working properly (i.e., end-stage renal disease or **nephropathy**).

DISORDERED EATING: Abnormal eating patterns characterized by starving, purging, bingeing, and/or other behaviors.

DISACCHARIDE: A double-unit sugar composed of two simple sugars, such as **sucrose** (**glucose** and **fructose**), maltose (two **glucose** units), and lactose (**glucose** and galactose).

EATING DISORDERS: Any type of **disordered eating** that has an official classification and name, such as **anorexia nervosa** or **bulimia nervosa**.

ECCENTRIC: The part of a muscle contraction with force development during the muscle-lengthening phase that is primarily responsible for **DOMS**.

ENDORPHINS: Brain **hormones** released in response to exercise, certain foods, and other external stimuli that positively alter mood. In exercisers, a "runner's high" caused by endorphin release results in feelings of euphoria and/or a "second wind."

ENDOTHELIAL DYSFUNCTION: Disturbed or altered blood flow through your blood vessels due to changes in the function of the endothelial (inner) layer of cells lining the vessels. It can result from intake of unhealthy foods, **hyperglycemia**, and other factors.

EXERCISE PHYSIOLOGIST: An exercise professional trained to understand the **metabolic** and other processes that occur in your body during exercise in health and disease.

FASTING: Going without eating overnight (for usually at least eight hours) or abstaining from food for an extended period at other times.

FAT: A nutrient found in foods primarily in the form of **triglycerides**; also refers to **adipose** tissue. The fat traveling in your circulation may also be called **lipids** and includes **triglycerides, free fatty acids**, and **cholesterol**.

FIBER: A collective term used to describe the indigestible **polysaccharides** that you get in your diet, both naturally from foods and from synthetic sources (e.g., fiber supplements).

FOOD GUIDE PYRAMID: A guide to supposedly balanced, healthy eating created by the U.S. Department of Agriculture to educate the public on proper nutritional habits.

FREE FATTY ACIDS: The breakdown products of **fat** that travel around your circulation bound to a blood protein called albumin. When delivered to muscles, free fatty acids can be picked up and used for energy or restored as **triglycerides** in your muscles, **adipose**, or liver.

FREE RADICALS: Compounds formed in cells during oxygen use that, if not controlled by **antioxidant** enzymes, can cause permanent (aging-related) damage to DNA in your cells and contribute to the formation of many **diabetic complications**.

FRUCTOSE: A simple sugar (**monosaccharide**) naturally occurring in fruit that has a relatively low **GI** value compared with most **refined sugars** or **glucose**.

GASTROPARESIS: A form of **autonomic neuropathy** that causes delayed emptying and absorption of ingested foods and fluids from the gut.

GLUCAGON: A **hormone** released by the alpha cells of the **pancreas** in response to exercise or **hypoglycemia** that acts by directly stimulating your liver to release more **glucose**.

GLUCOSE: One of the three simple **carbohydrates** classified as **monosaccharides**. Glucose is the primary carbohydrate available to all cells in your body via blood circulation and removed primarily either by **insulin**'s actions or by muscle contractions.

GLUTATHIONE: A compound found in foods or made by your body that is the main **antioxidant** enzyme found in all cells.

GLYCATED HEMOGLOBIN: A blood test that estimates your average **BG** level over the previous two to three months (also called "hemoglobin A_{1c}" or "**HbA_{1c}**"). To be in good control, your reading should be no higher than 7 percent and optimally less than 6.5 percent.

GLYCEMIA: The relative level of **glucose** in your circulation at any given time.

GLYCEMIC INDEX (GI): The system measuring the immediate effect that consumption of a particular food has on your **BG** levels. The more rapidly that **carbohydrates** are absorbed and show up as **glucose** in your bloodstream, the higher the glycemic spike and GI value a food has. On a scale from 1 to 100, **glucose** itself ranks 100.

GLYCEMIC LOAD (GL): A means of taking into account both the **GI** value and the quantity of **carbohydrates** that you eat using a scale of 0 (no **carbohydrate**) to 20 (high quantity and **glycemic** effect).

GLYCOGEN: The storage form of **glucose** in your body, whereby long chains of linked **glucose** molecules can be stored in your muscles and liver for later use.

HEART ATTACK: Permanent damage to the heart muscle resulting from a period of reduced blood flow (**ischemia**). It is usually the result of **coronary** artery blockage from **plaque** or a blood clot.

HEART DISEASE: Thickening of the inner walls of the **coronary** arteries caused by **plaque** formation that can reduce or block blood flow to the heart muscle.

HBA₁C: Abbreviation for **glycated hemoglobin**.

HDL: High-density lipoprotein, a subfraction of blood **cholesterol** (considered the "good" cholesterol) that works to remove excess cholesterol from your circulation.

HORMONE: A **protein-** or **lipid**-based compound made by the body and released by a gland into the circulation to affect another gland or tissue, such as when the **pancreas** releases **insulin** that causes **BG** to be taken up into cells to lower circulating levels of **glucose**.

HYPERGLYCEMIA: Any elevation in **BG** above what is normal for nondiabetic individuals after eating; usually 140 **mg/dl**.

HYPERINSULINEMIA: Abnormally high levels of circulating **insulin** secreted by your **pancreas** in an attempt to overcome your body's heightened state of **insulin resistance**.

HYPERTENSION: High blood pressure, defined as elevations in blood pressure readings above 140 and/or 90 for your higher and lower readings, respectively.

HYPOGLYCEMIA: A metabolic state clinically defined as any **BG** level at or lower than 65 **mg/dl**.

HYPOGLYCEMIC UNAWARENESS: A diabetic complication that results in an inability to sense when your **BG** level is too low, which can lead to dangerously low BG levels and unconsciousness. It is more common in individuals with **type 1 diabetes** than **type 2**.

HYPONATREMIA: Dangerously low levels of sodium in your bloodstream usually caused by excessive fluid intake during extended exercise, causing a range of symptoms from mild nausea to death; also called "water intoxication."

IMPAIRED GLUCOSE TOLERANCE (IGT): The inability of your body to respond with an adequate release of **insulin** following a large intake of **carbohydrate**. IGT is usually diagnosed with an oral **glucose** tolerance test in which you have to consume 75 grams of **glucose** and your BG levels are monitored for two or more hours afterward.

INCRETINS: The newest class of diabetic medications, derivatives of the venom of the Gila monster. They increase your insulin release, protect **beta cell** function, decrease your liver's production of **glucose**, and increase feelings of fullness after eating when injected.

INFLAMMATION: A process in which your body's white blood cells and other released chemicals attempt to protect you from infection and foreign substances, such as bacteria and viruses. Low-level, body-wide inflammation that may contribute to health complications, however, occurs in association with weight gain, **hypertension**, and **diabetes**.

INHALED INSULIN: A form of rapid-acting **insulin** that is inhaled into the lungs and absorbed through the walls of the lungs rather than injected under the skin.

INSULIN: A **hormone** produced by the **beta cells** of the **pancreas** that circulates in the bloodstream after its release in response to rising **BG** levels and causes insulin-sensitive tissues (muscles and **adipose**) to take up **glucose** into those cells for use.

INSULIN ANALOG: A slightly altered form of human **insulin** that has undergone synthetic substitution of a different amino acid or two somewhere in the normal insulin **protein** chain, causing it to be absorbed more rapidly (or more evenly, in the case of the basal analogs) from skin injection sites than normal synthetic human insulin.

INSULIN PUMPS: External devices about the size of a pager that you can utilize to dispense basal and bolus doses of **insulin** through tubing connected to a **subcutaneous** infusion site that must be rotated every two to three days; you control the dosing in response to your **BG** levels.

INSULIN RESISTANCE: A metabolic state whereby the **insulin** that your **pancreas** produces is less effective than it should be at stimulating your cells to take up **BG**, resulting in chronic **hyperinsulinemia** and/or **hyperglycemia**.

INSULIN SENSITIVITY: The relative ability of a given amount of circulating **insulin** to promote **glucose** uptake into cells around your body. Insulin action is increased by physical activity, low-**GI** diets, loss of **visceral fat**, reduced mental stress, certain medications, adequate sleep, and other factors.

INSULIN SENSITIZERS: Compounds, medications, or activities that have the capacity to increase the action of circulating insulin and increase its effectiveness at lowering **BG** levels.

INTERMEDIATE-ACTING INSULIN: Any type of injected **insulin** that provides coverage over a period of 8 to 12 hours, with a peak of **insulin** action at 3 to 4 hours, such as NPH.

INTERVAL TRAINING: Any form of exercise training that employs interspersed faster and slower periods of activity during training sessions.

ISCHEMIA: Reduced blood flow through the **coronary** arteries that supply the heart muscle due to blockage or constriction.

KETONES: Compounds derived from **free fatty acids** that circulate in the bloodstream when **hyperglycemia** is present and **insulin** is deficient.

KETOSIS: A potentially life-threatening **metabolic** acidosis caused by excessive **ketones** in the blood and dehydration; aka diabetic ketoacidosis or DKA.

LACTIC ACID SYSTEM: The body's second energy system, which provides energy from 30 seconds to two minutes into exercise by partially breaking down **carbohydrates** through **anaerobic** processes and forming lactic acid.

LDL: Low-density lipoproteins, the more damaging subfraction of **cholesterol** that circulates in your bloodstream and contributes to **plaque** formation.

LEPTIN: A **hormone** released by **adipose** cells that helps regulate food intake and body weight.

LIFESTYLE CHANGES: Permanent alterations in your normal behavior patterns with the intent of improving your health, primarily through increased physical activity, healthier food choices, stress reduction, cessation of smoking, and other healthy changes.

LIPID: Any fatty substance in your circulation, including **triglycerides**, **free fatty acids**, **cholesterol**, and more.

LONG-ACTING INSULIN: A synthetic **insulin** or **insulin analog** designed to be absorbed slowly and evenly over an extended time period (12 to 24 hours) to provide for your baseline (basal) **insulin** needs (e.g., Lantus or Levemir).

LSD TRAINING: Long, Slow Distance training: exercise training that is done for extended periods to build up your endurance base.

MAJOR DEPRESSIVE DISORDER: Major depression that leads to feelings of a profound and constant sense of hopelessness and despair and that can interfere with your ability to work, study, sleep, eat, and enjoy once-pleasurable activities.

MEGLITINIDES: A class of **oral diabetic medications** that are taken with meals specifically to promote additional **insulin** release to cover glycemic spikes.

METABOLIC: Related to your **metabolism**, which is the sum total of all processes occurring in your body that produce and use energy, create and break down tissues, and more.

METABOLISM: The sum total of all processes occurring in your body that produce and use energy, create and break down tissues, and more. It can be increased by gains in muscle mass.

METFORMIN: The generic name for the only currently FDA-approved **oral diabetic medication** in the **biguanide** class.

mg/dl: Milligrams per deciliter (of blood), the units designated for **BG** in the United States; other countries use **mM**, which is the equivalent of BG in mg/dl divided by 18 (e.g., 180 mg/dl equals 10 mM).

MIND-BODY CONNECTION: The special connection that appears to exist between your emotional health (thoughts and attitudes) and your physical well-being.

mM: millimolar, or millimoles per liter; units for the concentration of **BG** in most of the world with the notable exception of the United States (which uses **mg/dl**).

MONOSACCHARIDES: The simplest type of **carbohydrates**, including **glucose**, **fructose**, and galactose.

MONOUNSATURATED FAT: A type of **fat** in foods that is the most heart-healthy and least likely to cause **insulin resistance**, found in abundance in olive and canola oils.

MUSCLE FIBERS: Protein-based structures in muscle that interact to cause contraction and relaxation of muscles to accomplish any type of muscular work.

MUSCULAR ENDURANCE: The ability of your muscles to do a particular exercise for a given amount of time. In resistance work, how many sit-ups or pull-ups you can do in one minute is a measure of muscular endurance rather than **muscular strength**.

MUSCULAR STRENGTH: The maximal weight or resistance that your muscles can handle during one repetition of a task (i.e., **1-rep max**).

NEPHROPATHY: Damage to the kidneys due to chronic **hyperglycemia** that ultimately results in failure of the kidneys to filter blood properly and the need for a kidney transplant.

NEUROPATHY: Damage to nerves that can result in loss of feeling in your feet and hands, burning sensations in your extremities, **orthostatic hypotension**, **gastroparesis**, and more.

NON-WEIGHT-BEARING EXERCISES: Any physical activities that do not require you to carry the full brunt of your body weight on your legs or lower body, such as swimming, aqua aerobics, stationary cycling, and seated or arm-crank exercises.

NUTRITIONAL SUPPLEMENTS: Any dietary supplement taken with the intent of adding a nutrient to or supplementing the quantity of a nutrient in your diet, including **carbohydrates, protein, fat,** vitamins, minerals, **phytonutrients,** and other compounds.

OBESE: A clinical definition of your level of **overweight**; having a **BMI** of 30.0 or higher or being 120 percent or more of your ideal body weight.

OMEGA-3 FATTY ACIDS: One of two essential types of fatty acids in your diet. Omega-3s, including alpha-linolenic acid, EPA, and DHA, are anti-inflammatory and found mainly in fish.

OMEGA-6 FATTY ACIDS: Linoleic acid, the second essential fatty acid, which is found more in nuts and meats. This fatty acid can be pro-inflammatory when not balanced by omega-3s.

ORAL DIABETIC MEDICATIONS: Any of the prescription medications taken by mouth at least once daily that are utilized for the control of **BG,** such as **biguanides, sulfonylureas,** and **meglitinides.**

ORAL INSULIN: A form of insulin currently in clinical trials (awaiting FDA approval) that has been designed to withstand stomach acids and be absorbed by your body after you ingest it without being degraded like other **proteins.**

ORTHOSTATIC HYPOTENSION: Dizziness or fainting that occurs when you change bodily positions, such as going from sitting to standing, caused by **autonomic neuropathy.**

OSTEOPOROSIS: Thinning of your bones that can result in fractures and breaks.

OVERLOAD: An excessive workload placed on muscles during physical activity with the intent of causing gains in **muscular strength** and/or **muscular endurance.**

OVERUSE INJURIES: Joint and muscular injuries resulting from inflammation due to excessive **repetition** of a particular exercise or joint movement, such as rotator cuff tendonitis.

OVERUSE SYNDROME: Overstressing your body with repeated heavy workouts or extended exercise sessions to the point of causing more frequent colds, chronic tiredness, and **overuse injuries.**

OVERWEIGHT: A clinical definition of your level of excess body **fat;** normal lean adult **BMI** values range from 18.5 to less than 25.0 for adults, while overweight is characterized by a ratio of 25.0 to 29.9.

OXIDATIVE STRESS: Damage to your body's cells and tissues resulting from unchecked **free radicals** and one of the primary causes of diabetic complications and aging.

OXYGEN SYSTEM: Your body's third energy system, which utilizes oxygen to make **ATP** during rest and any physical activity lasting longer than two minutes.

PANCREAS: An organ located in the abdominal cavity behind the stomach that contains the **beta cells** that produce **insulin**, alpha cells that produce **glucagon**, and other cells that secrete digestive enzymes.

PEDOMETER: A small device about the size of a pager that counts the number of steps you take.

PERIPHERAL NEUROPATHY: Nerve damage affecting peripheral areas of your body, such as your hands and feet, resulting in shooting pains, burning sensations, and/or loss of feeling.

PERIPHERAL VASCULAR DISEASE (PVD): **Plaque** formation in arteries in your lower limbs, leading to restricted blood flow to legs and feet and commonly pain with exertion.

PHOSPHAGENS: A group of energy-releasing compounds (**ATP** and creatine phosphate) that act as your body's first energy system when exercise begins, up to 10 seconds of all-out effort.

PHYTONUTRIENTS: A class of phytochemicals with special functions in the body. Many of them have **antioxidant** properties and work synergistically with other such nutrients found with them in natural foods. Two examples are flavanols and procyanidins in dark chocolate.

PLAQUE: A deposit of fatty and other substances (including **LDL cholesterol**) in the inner wall of an artery as the result of an initial injury and **inflammation**, resulting in a narrowing of the artery at that point.

POLYMEAL: An alternate to the polypill, or taking multiple medications for all of your chronic health problems. The polymeal consists of heart-healthy and anti-inflammatory foods (like fish, wine, whole grains, and dark chocolate) that can improve your health and alleviate your chronic conditions naturally and without unpleasant side effects.

POLYSACCHARIDE: A **carbohydrate** containing a large number of **glucose** units bound together.

POLYUNSATURATED FAT: A type of dietary **fat** that is liquid at room temperature, found in most vegetable oils, nuts, and fish, and considered relatively heart healthy.

PREDIABETES: A health condition diagnosed with a **fasting BG** level of

100 to 125 **mg/dl** characterized by **insulin resistance** and **hyper-insulinemia**, with otherwise normal or nearly normal BG levels. Pre-diabetes can easily progress into **type 2 diabetes** once your body can't supply enough insulin to keep up with demand for it.

PROTEIN: The main nutrient found in meat and soy products, which, when consumed, your body breaks down into its constituent amino acids, which it then uses to build and repair muscles, **hormones**, enzymes, and other protein structures throughout your body.

QT INTERVAL: The point in your heart's contraction cycle when an abnormal beat that could be fatal is most likely to begin. A normal interval is 0.39 seconds in men and 0.41 seconds in women, but it is often prolonged in diabetic people in association with high **BG** levels, elevated **insulin** levels, and reduced **insulin sensitivity**.

RAPID-ACTING INSULIN ANALOG: Any of the synthetic **insulin analogs**, such as Humalog, NovoLog, and Apidra, which exert their main **glucose**-lowering effects within 30 minutes to three hours after a bolus injection and are used to provide insulin for meals and snacks.

REFINED CARBOHYDRATES: Any **carbohydrate**-based foods that have been highly processed, thereby stripping them of most or all of their essential nutrients, including white rice, white flour, white sugar, and more.

REFINED SUGARS: Simple **carbohydrates** that have been highly processed to the point of removing all nutrients, such as white table sugar, brown sugar, and corn syrup.

REPETITIONS (REPS): The number of times a resistance exercise (such as biceps curls) is repeated during each **set** (e.g., 8 to 12 reps per set).

RESISTANCE TRAINING: **Muscular strength** training done using resistance machines, free weights, dumbbells, or resistance bands to enhance the maximal power of the worked muscle(s). It is considered "progressive" if the resistances you use are periodically increased whenever you can complete more than the required number of **reps** per **set**.

RETINOL: The active form of vitamin A found in organ meats and fortified dairy products.

RETINOPATHY: A form of diabetic eye disease that results in the growth of abnormal vessels in the back of the eye (retina) that can break and bleed into the eye and block your vision.

RIB PRINCIPLE: An exercise-associated relaxation technique that stands for relaxation, imagination, and breathing.

SATURATED FAT: An unhealthy form of **fat** that is solid at room temperature, found mainly in meat, dairy products, and tropical oils (coconut, palm, and palm kernel), and contributes heavily to **plaque** formation and **heart disease**.

SELF-ESTEEM: A psychological term relating to the level of confidence and satisfaction you have in yourself, which can potentially be negatively affected by diabetes and excess weight.

SETS: The number of times a weight or resistance is lifted consecutively without stopping. Most **resistance training** workouts include one to three sets of 8 to 12 **reps** per set.

SILENT ISCHEMIA: A reduction in blood flow to the heart muscle that is painless and symptom-free due to diabetic **neuropathy** and that can result in an undetected or "silent" **heart attack**.

STATINS: A group of medications given to lower blood **cholesterol** or blood **fat** levels that may have negative effects on your ability to exercise without experiencing pain or fatigue.

STRESS HORMONES: Collectively, these are all of the hormones released by your body to prevent **hypoglycemia** and raise BG levels at rest and during exercise. They include **glucagon, adrenaline** (epinephrine), norepinephrine, growth hormone, and **cortisol**.

STROKE: Death of part of your brain caused by reduced blood flow through the carotid arteries (a stroke due to **ischemia**) or leakage from a brain blood vessel (a hemorrhagic stroke).

SUBCUTANEOUS: Refers to the tissue layer immediately under the surface of the skin, such as subcutaneous **fat**.

SUCROSE: White table sugar, a **disaccharide** comprised of **glucose** and **fructose**.

SUGAR ALCOHOLS: Derivatives of sugar, such as sorbitol, that are put in foods to make them "sugar free," but that contain almost as many calories. Some may be absorbed more slowly than sugar or may not be completely absorbed at all, and many can cause diarrhea if eaten in excess.

SULFONYLUREAS: The first developed class of **oral diabetic medications**, which act by stimulating your **beta cells** to make and release more **insulin** to lower **BG** levels.

TALK TEST: An informal test used to determine if you are exercising too intensely. You should be able to carry on a conversation with someone else during an activity; if you can't talk freely due to heavy breathing, slow down, as you are working harder than needed.

TARGET HEART RATES: Calculated heart-rate ranges used to monitor exercise intensity based on age and **aerobic** conditioning goals. These rates are most commonly a percentage (e.g., 70 to 85 percent) of your maximum heart-rate increase above resting levels.

TNF-ALPHA: Tumor necrosis factor–alpha, a compound believed to be involved in the development of the low-level system **inflammation** present in diabetes and insulin-resistant states and in the progression of other immune functions.

TRACE MINERALS: Minerals needed by your body in minute quantities, such as iron, fluoride, and iodine. Other minerals, such as calcium, sodium, and potassium, are more abundant in your body and in the foods that you eat and do not qualify as "trace" minerals.

TRANS FAT: A form of dietary **fat** usually created by food manufacturing practices that cause the **fat** to become more **saturated**, thus more potentially damaging to arteries. You should try to consume as little of this **fat** as possible to limit your **heart disease** risk.

TRIGLYCERIDES: The main type of **fat** in foods that you eat, as well as the main storage form for **fat** in your muscles and **adipose** tissues.

TYPE 1 DIABETES: An autoimmune disease in which the body's own immune cells attack and destroy the **beta cells** of the **pancreas**, rendering them unable to make much or any **insulin**. Individuals with type 1 diabetes must inject insulin for the rest of their lives.

TYPE 1.5 DIABETES: A new term being used to describe "double diabetes," or a form of **diabetes** that has characteristics of both **type 1 (autoimmunity)** and **type 2 (insulin resistance)**.

TYPE 2 DIABETES: A disease characterized by a heightened state of **insulin resistance** in combination with the loss of at least some of **beta cell** insulin production, resulting in **hyperglycemia** and abnormal blood **fat** (i.e., **cholesterol** and **triglyceride**) levels.

VISCERAL FAT: Body **fat** stored deep within the abdominal region that is more metabolically active than most **adipose** tissue and is associated with **insulin resistance** and **type 2 diabetes**.

WAIST CIRCUMFERENCE: The measurement around your waist at the level of your umbilicus (belly button). Elevated waist circumferences are closely associated with **metabolic** abnormalities, including **hypertension**, **type 2 diabetes**, and **cardiovascular disease**.

WAIST-TO-HIP RATIO (WHR): The relative measurements of your **waist circumference** and your hip circumference at its widest point. A high

WHR has been associated with **abdominal obesity** and other **metabolic** disorders.

WARMUP: A five- to ten-minute period of easier exercise done at the start of more intense physical activity that serves to increase circulation to muscles and warm up joints.

Suggested Reading

Becker, Gretchen. *The First Year—Type 2 Diabetes: An Essential Guide for the Newly Diagnosed.* New York: Marlowe & Company, 2001.

Brand-Miller, Jennie, et al. *The New Glucose Revolution.* New York: Marlowe & Company, 2003.

Bricklin, Mark, and Linda Konner. *Prevention's Your Perfect Weight: The Diet-Free Weight-Loss Method Developed by the World's Leading Health Magazine.* Emmaus, PA: Rodale Press, 1995.

Colberg, Sheri. *Diabetes-Free Kids: A Take-Charge Plan for Preventing and Treating Type 2 Diabetes in Children.* New York: Avery, 2005.

Colberg, Sheri. *The Diabetic Athlete: Prescriptions for Exercise and Sports.* Champaign, IL: Human Kinetics, 2001.

Barnes, Darryl. *Action Plan for Diabetes: Your Guide to Controlling Blood Sugar.* Champaign, IL: Human Kinetics, 2004

Gaesser, Glenn. *Big Fat Lies: The Truth About Your Weight and Your Health.* Carlsbad, CA: Gürze Books, 2002.

Hayes, Charlotte. *The "I Hate to Exercise" Book for People with Diabetes.* Alexandria, VA: American Diabetes Association, 2000.

Hornsby, W. Guyton, ed. *The Fitness Book: For People with Diabetes (A Project of the American Diabetes Association Council on Exercise).* Alexandria, VA: American Diabetes Association, 1994.

Joseph, James, Daniel Nadeau, and Anne Underwood. *The Color Code: A Revolutionary Eating Plan for Optimal Health.* New York: Hyperion, 2003.

Nathan, David, and Linda Delahanty. *Beating Diabetes (A Harvard Medical School Book).* New York: McGraw-Hill, 2005.

Peters, Anne. *Conquering Diabetes: A Cutting-Edge, Comprehensive Program for Prevention and Treatment.* New York: Hudson Street Press, 2005.

Price, Joan. *The Anytime, Anywhere Exercise Book.* Avon, MA: Adams Media Corporation, 2003.

Ruderman, Neil, ed. *Handbook of Exercise in Diabetes.* Alexandria, VA: American Diabetes Association, 2002.

Scheiner, Gary. *Think Like a Pancreas: A Practical Guide to Managing Diabetes with Insulin.* New York: Marlowe & Company, 2004.

Schlosberg, Suzanne, and Liz Neporent. *Weight Training for Dummies.* New York: Hungry Minds (Wiley), 1997.

Warshaw, Hope. *Guide to Healthy Restaurant Eating.* Boston, MA: McGraw-Hill/Contemporary Books, 2002.

Selected References

Introduction

Centers for Disease Control and Prevention. 2000. National Diabetes Fact Sheet: General information and national estimates on diabetes in the United States, 2000. Retrieved from http://www.cdc.gov/diabetes/pubs/estimates.htm.

Hu, G., P. Jousilahti, N. C. Barengo, et al. 2005. Physical activity, cardiovascular risk factors, and mortality among Finnish adults with diabetes. *Diabetes Care* 28:799–805.

Narayan, K., J. Boyle, T. Thompson, et al. 2003. Lifetime risk for diabetes mellitus in the United States. *Journal of the American Medical Association* 290:1884–90.

Stevens, J., J. Cai, K. Evenson, and R. Thomas. 2002. Fitness and fatness as predictors of mortality from all causes and from cardiovascular disease in men and women in the Lipid Research Clinics Study. *American Journal of Epidemiology* 156:832–41.

Whiteley, L., S. Padmanabhan, D. Hole, et al. 2005. Should diabetes be considered a coronary heart disease risk equivalent? *Diabetes Care* 28:1588–93.

Step 1

Aas, A. M., I. Bergstad, P. M. Thorsby, et al. 2005. An intensified lifestyle intervention programme may be superior to insulin treatment in poorly controlled type 2 diabetic patients on oral hypoglycaemic agents: Results of a feasibility study. *Diabetic Medicine* 22:316–22.

Almond, C. S., A. Y. Shin, E. B. Fortescue, et al. 2005. Hyponatremia among runners in the Boston Marathon. *New England Journal of Medicine* 352:1550–56.

American College of Sports Medicine. 2000. Exercise and type 2 diabetes. *Medicine & Science in Sports & Exercise* 32:1345–60.

Berggren, J., M. Hulver, G. L. Dohm, and J. Houmard. 2004. Weight loss and exercise: Implications for muscle lipid metabolism and insulin action. *Medicine & Science in Sports & Exercise* 36:1191–95.

Borghouts, L., and H. Keizer. 2000. Exercise and insulin sensitivity: A review. *International Journal of Sports Medicine* 21:1–12.

Bruce, C., and J. Hawley. 2004. Improvements in insulin resistance with aerobic exercise training: A lipocentric approach. *Medicine & Science in Sports & Exercise* 36:1196–1201.

Bruunsgaard, H. 2005. Physical activity and modulation of systemic low-level inflammation. *Journal of Leukocyte Biology.* 78:1–17.

Cox, K. L., V. Burke, A. R. Morton, et al. 2004. Independent and additive effects of energy restriction and exercise on glucose and insulin concentrations in sedentary overweight men. *American Journal of Clinical Nutrition* 80:308–16.

Cuff, D. J., G. S. Meneilly, A. Martin, et al. 2003. Effective exercise modality to reduce insulin resistance in women with type 2 diabetes. *Diabetes Care* 26:2977–82.

Dela, F., K. J. Mikines, J. J. Larsen, and H. Galbo. 1999. Glucose clearance in trained skeletal muscle during maximal insulin with superimposed exercise. *Journal of Applied Physiology* 87:2059–67.

Dela, F., M. E. von Linstow, K. J. Mikines, and H. Galbo. 2004. Physical training may enhance beta-cell function in type 2 diabetes. *American Journal of Physiology* 287:E1024–31.

Dunstan, D. W., R. M. Daly, N. Owen, et al. 2002. High-intensity resistance training improves glycemic control in older patients with type 2 diabetes. *Diabetes Care* 25:1729–36.

Ebeling, P., H. A. Koistinen, and V. A. Koivisto. 1998. Insulin-independent glucose transport regulates insulin sensitivity. *FEBS Letters* 436:301–303.

Eriksson, J. W., U. Smith, F. Waagstein, et al. 1999. Glucose turnover and adipose tissue lipolysis are insulin-resistant in healthy relatives of type 2 diabetic patients: Is cellular insulin resistance a secondary phenomenon? *Diabetes* 48:1572–78.

Giannopoulou, I., L. L. Ploutz-Synder, R. Carhart, et al. 2005. Exercise is required for visceral fat loss in postmenopausal women with type 2 diabetes. *Journal of Clinical Endocrinology and Metabolism* 90:1511–18.

Hawley, J. A. 2004. Exercise as a therapeutic intervention for the prevention and treatment of insulin resistance. *Diabetes/Metabolism Research and Reviews* 20:383–93.

Hu, F. B., R. J. Sigal, J. W. Rich-Edwards, et al. 1999. Walking compared with vigorous physical activity and risk of type 2 diabetes in women: A prospective study. *Journal of the American Medical Association* 282:1433–39.

Ibañez, J., M. Izquierdo, I. Argüelles, et al. 2005. Twice-weekly progressive resistance training decreases abdominal fat and improves insulin sensitivity in older men with type 2 diabetes. *Diabetes Care* 28:662–67.

Ishii, T., T. Yamakita, T. Sato, et al. 1998. Resistance training improves insulin sensitivity in NIDDM subjects without altering maximal oxygen uptake. *Diabetes Care* 21:1351–55.

King, D., G. Dalsky, W. Clutter, et al. 1988. Effects of lack of exercise on insulin secretion and action in trained subjects. *American Journal of Physiology* 254:E537–42.

Knowler, W. C., E. Barrett-Connor, S. E. Fowler, et al. 2002. Reduction in the incidence of type 2 diabetes with lifestyle intervention or metformin. *New England Journal of Medicine* 346:393–403.

Manson, J. E., E. B. Rimm, M. J. Stampfer, et al. 1991. Physical activity and incidence of non-insulin-dependent diabetes mellitus in women. *Lancet* 338:774–78.

Mayers, D. 2005. Is dieting bad for you? Experts debate whether losing weight is the wrong prescription for better health. *Diabetes Health* 14:50–52, 54–55.

McCartney, N. 1999. Acute responses to resistance training and safety. *Medicine & Science in Sports & Exercise* 31:31–37.

Nagano, M., Y. Kai, B. Zou, et al. 2004. The contribution of cardiorespiratory fitness and visceral fat to risk factors in Japanese patients with impaired glucose tolerance and type 2 diabetes mellitus. *Metabolism* 53:644–49.

Peres, S. B., S. M. de Moraes, C. E. Costa, et al. 2005. Endurance exercise training increases insulin responsiveness in isolated adipocytes through IRS/PI3-Kinase/Akt pathway. *Journal of Applied Physiology* 98:1037–43.

Petersen, A. M., and B. K. Pedersen. 2005. The anti-inflammatory effect of exercise. *Journal of Applied Physiology* 98:1154–62.

Poirier, P., S. Mawhinney, L. Gondin, et al. 2001. Prior meal enhances the plasma glucose lowering effect of exercise in type 2 diabetes. *Medicine & Science in Sports & Exercise* 33:1259–64.

Savage, D. B., K. F. Petersen, and G. I. Shulman. 2005. Mechanisms of insulin resistance in humans and possible links with inflammation. *Hypertension* 45:828–33.

Sullivan, P. W., E. H. Morrato, V. Ghushchyan, et al. 2005. Obesity, inactivity, and the prevalence of diabetes and diabetes-related cardiovascular comorbidities in the U.S., 2000–2002. *Diabetes Care* 28:1599–1603.

Tuomilehto, J., J. Lindstrom, J. G. Eriksson, et al. 2001. Prevention of type 2 diabetes mellitus by changes in lifestyle among subjects with impaired glucose tolerance. *New England Journal of Medicine* 344:1343–50.

Wang, Y., E. B. Rimm, M. J. Stampfer, et al. 2005. Comparison of abdominal adiposity and overall obesity in predicting risk of type 2 diabetes among men. *American Journal of Clinical Nutrition* 81:555–63.

Wing, R., and J. Hill. 2001. Successful weight loss maintenance. *Annual Reviews in Nutrition* 21:323–41.

Step 2

American College of Sports Medicine. 2000. Exercise and type 2 diabetes. *Medicine & Science in Sports & Exercise* 32:1345–60.

Di Loreto, C., C. Fanelli, P. Lucidi, et al. 2005. Make your diabetic patients walk: Long-term impact of different amounts of physical activity on type 2 diabetes. *Diabetes Care* 28:1295–1302.

Dunstan, D. W., R. M. Daly, N. Owen, et al. 2005. Home-based resistance training is not sufficient to maintain improved glycemic control following supervised training in older individuals with type 2 diabetes. *Diabetes Care* 28:3–9.

Hu, F. B., R. J. Sigal, J. W. Rich-Edwards, et al. 1999. Walking compared with vigorous physical activity and risk of type 2 diabetes in women: A prospective study. *Journal of the American Medical Association* 282:1433–39.

Hultquist, C. N., C. Albright, and D. L. Thompson. 2005. Comparison of walking recommendations in previously inactive women. *Medicine & Science in Sports & Exercise* 37:676–83.

Sigal, R. J., G. P. Kenny, D. H. Wasserman, et al. 2004. Physical activity/exercise and type 2 diabetes. *Diabetes Care* 27:2518–38.

Simoneau, J. A., J. H. Veerkamp, L. P. Turcotte, D. E. Kelley. 1999. Markers of capacity to utilize fatty acids in human skeletal muscle: relation to insulin resistance and obesity and effects of weight loss. *FASEB Journal* 13:2051–60.

Step 3

American College of Sports Medicine. 2000. Exercise and type 2 diabetes. *Medicine & Science in Sports & Exercise* 32:1345–60.

American College of Sports Medicine. 1998. The recommended quantity and quality of exercise for developing and maintaining cardiorespiratory and muscular fitness, and flexibility in healthy adults. *Medicine & Science in Sports & Exercise* 30:975–91.

Bemben, D. A., N. L. Fetters, M. G. Bemben, et al. 2000. Musculoskeletal responses to high- and low-intensity resistance training in early postmenopausal women. *Medicine & Science in Sports & Exercise* 32:1949–57.

Bergman, B. C., G. E. Butterfield, E. E. Wolfel, et al. 1999. Muscle net glucose uptake and glucose kinetics after endurance training in men. *American Journal of Physiology* 277:E81–92.

de Vreede, P. L., M. M. Samson, N. L. van Meeteren, et al. 2005. Functional-task exercise versus resistance strength exercise to improve daily function in older women: a randomized, controlled trial. *Journal of the American Geriatrics Society* 53:2–10.

Herriott, M. T., S. R. Colberg, H. K. Parson, et al. 2004. Effects of eight weeks of flexibility and resistance training in older adults with type 2 diabetes. *Diabetes Care* 27:2988–89.

Houmard, J. A., C. J. Tanner, C. A. Slentz, et al. 2004. Effect of the volume and intensity of exercise training on insulin sensitivity. *Journal of Applied Physiology* 96:101–6.

Kemmler, W. K., D. Lauber, K. Engelke, and J. Weineck. 2004. Effects of single- vs. multiple-set resistance training on maximum strength and body composition in trained postmenopausal women. *Journal of Strength and Conditioning Research* 18:689–94.

Kubukeli, Z. N., T. D. Noakes, and S. C. Dennis. 2002. Training techniques to improve endurance exercise performances. *Sports Medicine* 32:489–509.

Vincent, K. R., R. W. Braith, R. A. Feldman, et al. 2002. Resistance exercise and physical performance in adults aged 60 to 83. *Journal of the American Geriatrics Society* 50:1100–07.

Willey, K. A., and M. A. Fiatarone Singh. 2003. Battling insulin resistance in elderly obese people with type 2 diabetes: Bring on the heavy weights. *Diabetes Care* 26:1580–88.

Winett, R. A., J. R. Wojcik, L. D. Fox, et al. 2003. Effects of low volume resistance and cardiovascular training on strength and aerobic capacity in unfit men and women: A demonstration of a threshold model. *Journal of Behavioral Medicine* 26:183–95.

Step 4

American Diabetes Association. 2004. Clinical practice recommendations: Nutrition principles and recommendations in diabetes. *Diabetes Care* 27:S36–46.

Boden, G., K. Sargrad, C. Homko, et al. 2005. Effect of a low-carbohydrate diet on appetite, blood glucose levels, and insulin resistance in obese patients with type 2 diabetes. *Annals of Internal Medicine* 142:403–11.

Brand-Miller, J., S. Hayne, P. Petocz, and S. Colagiuri. 2003. Low–glycemic index diets in the management of diabetes: A meta-analysis of randomized control trials. *Diabetes Care* 26:2261–67.

Farshchi, H. R., M. A. Taylor, and I. A. Macdonald. 2005. Deleterious effects of omitting breakfast on insulin sensitivity and fasting lipid profiles in healthy lean women. *American Journal of Clinical Nutrition* 81:388–96.

Foster-Powell, K., S. Holt, and J. Brand-Miller. 2002. International table of glycemic index and glycemic load values: 2002. *American Journal of Clinical Nutrition* 76:5–56.

Franco, D. H., L. Bonneux, C. de Laet, et al. 2004. The polymeal: A more natural, safer, and probably tastier (than the polypill) strategy to reduce cardiovascular disease by more than 75 percent. *British Medical Journal* 329:1447–50.

Giannopoulou, I., L. L. Ploutz-Synder, R. Carhart, et al. 2005. Exercise is required for visceral fat loss in postmenopausal women with type 2 diabetes. *Journal of Clinical Endocrinology and Metabolism* 90:1511–18.

Goudswaard, A., R. Stalk, H. de Valk, and G. Rutten. 2003. Improving glycaemic control in patients with type 2 diabetes mellitus without insulin therapy. *Diabetic Medicine* 20:540–44.

Grassi, D., C. Lippi, S. Necozione, et al. 2005. Short-term administration of dark chocolate is followed by a significant increase in insulin sensitivity and a decrease in blood pressure in healthy persons. *American Journal of Clinical Nutrition* 81:611–14.

Jayaprakasam, B., S. K. Vareed, L. K. Olson, et al. 2005. Insulin secretion by bioactive anthocyanins and anthocyanidins present in fruits. *Journal of Agricultural and Food Chemistry* 53:28–31.

Lee, S., R. Hudson, K. Kilpatrick, et al. 2005. Caffeine ingestion is associated with reductions in glucose uptake independent of obesity and type 2 diabetes before and after exercise training. *Diabetes Care* 28:566–72.

Liu, R. 2003. Health benefits of fruit and vegetables are from additive and synergistic combinations of phytochemicals. *American Journal of Clinical Nutrition* 78:517S–520S.

Lovejoy, J. 2002. The influence of dietary fat on insulin resistance. *Current Diabetes Reports* 2:435–40.

Ma, Y., B. Olendzki, D. Chiriboga, et al. 2005. Association between dietary carbohydrates and body weight. *American Journal of Epidemiology* 161:359–67.

Qi, L., E. Rimm, S. Liu, et al. 2005. Dietary glycemic index, glycemic load, cereal fiber, and plasma adiponectin concentration in diabetic men. *Diabetes Care* 28:1022–28.

Rizkalla, S., L. Taghrid, M. Laromiguiere, et al. 2004. Improved plasma glucose control, whole-body glucose utilization, and lipid profile on a low-glycemic index diet in type 2 diabetic men. *Diabetes Care* 27:1866–72.

Sargrad, K. R., C. Homko, M. Mozzoli, and G. Boden. 2005. Effect of high protein vs. high carbohydrate intake on insulin sensitivity, body weight, hemo-globin A1c, and blood pressure in patients with type 2 diabetes mellitus. *Journal of the American Dietetic Association* 105:573–80.

Trichopoulou, A., T. Costacou, C. Bamia, et al. 2003. Adherence to a Mediter-ranean diet and survival in a Greek population. *New England Journal of Medicine* 348:2599–2608.

Willett, W., J. Manson, and S. Liu. 2002. Glycemic index, glycemic load, and risk of type 2 diabetes. *American Journal of Clinical Nutrition* 76:274S–280S.

Zemel, M. B., J. Richards, S. Mathis, et al. 2005. Dairy augmentation of total and central fat loss in obese subjects. *International Journal of Obesity* 29:391–97.

Step 5

Clark, M. 2004. Is weight loss a realistic goal of treatment in type 2 diabetes? The implications of restraint theory. *Patient Counseling and Education* 53:277–83.

Egede, L. E. 2005. Effect of comorbid chronic diseases on prevalence and odds of depression in adults with diabetes. *Psychometric Medicine* 67:46–51.

Koppes, L. L., J. M. Dekker, H. F. Hendriks, et al. 2005. Moderate alcohol con-sumption lowers the risk of type 2 diabetes: A meta-analysis of prospective observational studies. *Diabetes Care* 28:719–25.

Krein, S. L., M. Heisler, J. D. Piette, et al. 2005. The effect of chronic pain on diabetes patients' self-management. *Diabetes Care* 28:65–70.

Kull, M. 2002. The relationships between physical activity, health status and psychological well-being of fertility-aged women. *Scandinavian Journal of Medicine & Science in Sports* 12:241–47.

Su, F., Y. Y. Chang, H. H. Pai, et al. 2004. Infusion of beta-endorphin improves insulin resistance in fructose-fed rats. *Hormone & Metabolism Research* 36:571–77.

Timonen, M., M. Laakso, J. Jokelainen, et al. 2005. Insulin resistance and depression: cross sectional study. *British Medical Journal* 330:17–18.

Whitmer, R. A., E. P. Gunderson, E. Barrett-Connor, et al. 2005. Obesity in mid-dle age and future risk of dementia: a 27-year longitudinal population-based study. *British Medical Journal* 330:1360–64.

Zhang, X., S. L. Norris, E. W. Gregg, et al. 2005. Depressive symptoms and mor-tality among persons with and without diabetes. *American Journal of Epidemi-ology* 161:652–60.

Step 6

Buse, J. B., R. R. Henry, J. Han, et al. 2004. Effects of exenatide (exendin-4) on glycemic control over 30 weeks in sulfonylurea-treated patients with type 2 diabetes. *Diabetes Care* 27:2628–35.

Chausmer, A. 1998. Zinc, insulin and diabetes. *Journal of the American College of Nutrition* 17:109–15.

Cheng, H. H., M. H. Lai, W. C. Hou, and C. L. Huang. 2004. Antioxidant effects of chromium supplementation with type 2 diabetes mellitus and eug-lycemic subjects. *Journal of Agricultural and Food Chemistry* 52:1385–89.

Chiu, K., A. Chu, V. Go, and M. Saad. 2004. Low vitamin D worsens beta cell function. *American Journal of Clinical Nutrition* 79:820–25.

Cook, M. N., C. J. Girman, P. P. Stein, et al. 2005. Glycemic control continues to deteriorate after sulfonylureas are added to metformin among patients with type 2 diabetes. *Diabetes Care* 28:995–1000.

Cusi, K., S. Cukier, R. DeFronzo, et al. 2001. Vanadyl sulfate improves hepatic and muscle insulin sensitivity in type 2 diabetes. *Journal of Clinical Endocrinology and Metabolism* 86:1410–17.

Dailey, G., J. Rosenstock, R. G. Moses, et al. 2004. Insulin glulisine [Apidra] provides improved glycemic control in patients with type 2 diabetes. *Diabetes Care* 27:2363–68.

Farvid, M. S., F. Siassi, M. Jalali, et al. 2004. The impact of vitamin and/or mineral supplementation on lipid profiles in type 2 diabetes. *Diabetes Research and Clinical Practice* 65:21–28.

Hallsten, K., K. A. Virtanen, F. Lonnqvist, et al. 2002. Rosiglitazone but not metformin enhances insulin- and exercise-stimulated skeletal muscle glucose uptake in patients with newly diagnosed type 2 diabetes. *Diabetes* 51:3479–85.

Joy, S. V., P. T. Rodgers, A. C. Scates. 2005. Incretin mimetics as emerging treatment for type 2 diabetes. *Annals of Pharmacotherapy* 39:110–18.

Kendall, D. M., M. C. Riddle, J. Rosenstock, et al. 2005. Effects of exenatide (exendin-4) on glycemic control over 30 weeks in patients with type 2 diabetes treated with metformin and a sulfonylurea. *Diabetes Care* 28:1083–91.

Khan, A., M. Safdar, M. M. Ali Khan, et al. 2003. Cinnamon improves glucose and lipids of people with type 2 diabetes. *Diabetes Care* 26:3215–18.

Larsen, J., F. Dela, S. Madsbad, et al. 1999. Interaction of sulfonylureas and exercise on glucose homeostasis in type 2 diabetic patients. *Diabetes Care* 22:1647–54.

Lee, D. H., A. R. Folsom, L. Harnack, et al. 2004. Does supplemental vitamin C increase cardiovascular disease risk in women with diabetes? *American Journal of Clinical Nutrition* 80:1194–1200.

Rabinovitz, H., A. Friedensohn, A. Leibovitz, et al. 2004. Effect of chromium supplementation on blood glucose and lipid levels in type 2 diabetes mellitus elderly patients. *International Journal for Vitamin and Nutrition Research* 74:178–82.

Raskin, P., E. Allen, P. Hollander, et al. 2005. Initiating insulin therapy in type 2 diabetes: a comparison of biphasic and basal insulin analogs. *Diabetes Care* 28:260–65.

Rave, K., S. Bott, L. Heinemann, et al. 2005. Time-action profile of inhaled insulin in comparison with subcutaneously injected insulin lispro and regular human insulin. *Diabetes Care* 28:1077–82.

Reusch, J. E., J. G. Regensteiner, P. A. Watson. 2003. Novel actions of thiazolidinediones on vascular function and exercise capacity. *American Journal of Medicine* 115:69S–74S.

Ruhe, R., and R. McDonald. 2001. Use of antioxidant nutrients in the prevention and treatment of type 2 diabetes. *Journal of the American College of Nutrition* 20:363S–368S.

Ryan, E., S. Imes, and C. Wallace. 2001. Short-term intensity insulin therapy in newly diagnosed type 2 diabetes. *Diabetes Care* 27:1028–32.

Yeh, G., D. Eisenberg, T. Kaptchuk, and R. Phillips. 2003. Systematic review of herbs and dietary supplements for glycemic control in diabetes. *Diabetes Care* 26:1277–94.

Step 7

Deshpande, A. D., E. A. Baker, S. L. Lovegreen, R. C. Brownson. 2005. Environmental correlates of physical activity among individuals with diabetes in the rural Midwest. *Diabetes Care* 28:1012–18.

de Vreede, P. L., M. M. Samson, N. L. van Meeteren, et al. 2004. Functional tasks exercise versus resistance exercise to improve daily function in older women: A feasibility study. *Archives of Physical Medicine and Rehabilitation* 85:1952–61.

Grossman, M. D., A. L. Stewart. 2003. "You aren't going to get better by just sitting around": Physical activity perceptions, motivations, and barriers in adults 75 years of age or older. *American Journal of Geriatric Cardiology* 12:33–37.

Lerman, I., L. Lozano, A. R. Villa, et al. 2004. Psychosocial factors associated with poor diabetes self-care management in a specialized center in Mexico City. *Biomedicine and Pharmacotherapy* 58:566–70.

Park, H., Y. Hong, H. Lee, E. Ha, and Y. Sung. 2004. Individuals with type 2 diabetes and depressive symptoms exhibited lower adherence with self-care. *Journal of Clinical Epidemiology* 57:978–84.

Seefeldt, V., R. M. Malina, and M. A. Clark. 2002. Factors affecting levels of physical activity in adults. *Sports Medicine* 32:143–68.

Acknowledgments

WITHOUT THE ASSISTANCE of many interested parties, the creation of this book would not have been possible, and my heartfelt thanks go to all of them. They should feel proud to be part of a book that can potentially help the multitude of people with diabetes worldwide to live longer and healthier lives.

First and foremost, I owe a world of thanks to my literary agent, Linda Konner, for her belief in the concept behind this book and for supporting me in my quest to put my passion for exercise into words that anyone with diabetes can live better by.

Next, my heartfelt gratitude goes to Patrick Ochs, my talented brother-in-law, who created the magnificent line drawings and illustrations for this book with the greatest of ease. If only my artistic talent were as fine-tuned as his. . . .

I am additionally grateful to Dr. Anne Peters, who believed in the worthiness of this topic enough to compose its foreword. Her willingness to participate, along with her own efforts in conquering diabetes, can only help spread the word on how everyone can live well despite diabetes.

I would also like to thank Dr. Aaron Vinik, a world-renowned diabetologist and neuropathy specialist whom I am lucky to have as my research collaborator and mentor at the Strelitz Diabetes Institutes, for his insightful review of the diabetic medications discussed in step 6 of this book. The fact that he can find the time to do anything more (such as reviewing my writing) than he already does always amazes me.

Finally, I would also like to acknowledge all of the hard-working individuals at Marlowe & Company who have helped in the creation of this book. I am particularly in debt to Matthew Lore, my publisher, who believes in this concept as much as I do and offered invaluable advice on how to share my knowledge more effectively with my readers, and to Peter Jacoby, his competent and hard-working assistant, as well as to all of the other devoted individuals involved with my book at Marlowe from start to finish.

My sincere gratitude extends to all of you.

Index

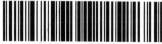

Made in the USA
Lexington, KY
07 January 2013